Thrive in Immunology

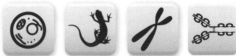

Other titles in the Thrive in Bioscience Series

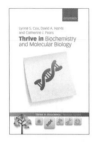

Thrive in Biochemistry
and Molecular Biology

Lynne S. Cox,
David A. Harris,
and Catherine J. Pears

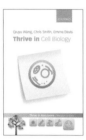

Thrive in Cell Biology

Qiuyu Wang, Chris Smith,
and Emma Davis

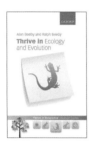

Thrive in Ecology and Evolution

Alan Beeby and Ralph Beeby

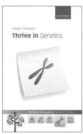

Thrive in Genetics

Alison Thomas

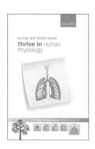

Thrive in Human Physiology

Ian Kay and Gethin Evans

Thrive in Immunology

Anne C. Cunningham
Associate Professor, PAPRSB Institute of Health Sciences,
Universiti Brunei Darussalam

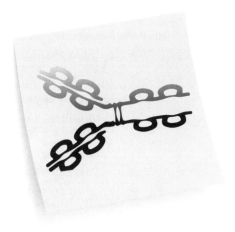

Thrive in Bioscience | Revision Guides

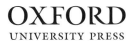

OXFORD
UNIVERSITY PRESS

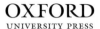

OXFORD
UNIVERSITY PRESS

Great Clarendon Street, Oxford, OX2 6DP,
United Kingdom

Oxford University Press is a department of the University of Oxford.
It furthers the University's objective of excellence in research, scholarship,
and education by publishing worldwide. Oxford is a registered trade mark of
Oxford University Press in the UK and in certain other countries

Published in the United States of America by Oxford University Press
198 Madison Avenue, New York, NY 10016, United States of America

British Library Cataloguing in Publication Data

Data available

Library of Congress Control Number: 2015955921

ISBN 978–0–19–964297–7

Printed in Great Britain by
Bell & Bain Ltd., Glasgow

Contents

Four steps to exam success

1 Review the facts

This book is designed to help you learn quickly and effectively:

- Information is set out in bullet points, making it easy to digest
- Clear, uncluttered illustrations illuminate what is said in the text
- Key concept panels indicate the essential learning points for a topic

2 Check your understanding

- Try the questions in each chapter and online multiple-choice questions to reinforce your learning
- Use the flashcard glossary to master the essential terms and phrases

3 Take note of extra advice

- Look out for hints for getting those precious extra marks in exams

4 Go the extra mile

- Explore other sources of information—including immunology textbooks—to take your knowledge and understanding one step further

Go to the Online Resource Centre for more resources to support your learning, including:

- Online quizzes, with feedback
- A flashcard glossary, to help you master the essential terminology

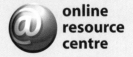
online
resource
centre

www.oxfordtextbooks.co.uk/orc/thrive/

Using this guide

This book is designed to be an *aide memoire* and a quick check-up source rather than an authoritative text. You will need to have revised material from your lecture notes, text books and recommended reading lists in order to get full value from this book. It aims to include core material that is central to an understanding of immunology. However, courses differ, so not all the material here may be covered in your course, and there may be bits that aren't included here that you do need to know about. It is also worth checking out the other revision guides in this series on, for example, cell biology and genetics, according to your own course requirements.

The material is arranged into related sections, though the book does cross-reference between sections where relevant. Important terms are highlighted in bold and have a definition in the Glossary at the back of the book. Sometimes it can be hard to remember all the points about a topic, so the topics are broken down into smaller chunks to make revision easier.

Exam technique

When answering **short questions**, ensure that your answer is concise and precise, containing all the information required but no waffle or irrelevant information. In some cases, it is OK to use bullet points, but not in others, so make sure you choose a format appropriate to your own University's exams. Although exam styles vary, examiners will always appreciate scientific accuracy, relevance and logical argument.

There are some sample exam questions included in the book with hints (worked answers aren't given as the text itself is in essence the answer), and there are multiple choice tests online linked to each section of the book, so you can check your progress in revision.

 www.oxfordtextbooks.co.uk/orc/thrive/

Using this guide

For **multiple choice questions**, try to come up with the correct answer first, then check the answers given—be particularly careful when you have to identify correct combinations of answers. For example:

Which of the following is true about CD antigens?
  i) They are only found on leukocytes
  ii) They are all cell surface molecules
  iii) They can be identified by specific monoclonal antibodies
  iv) They all have similar functions
  v) They can help to phenotype leukocytes

Answers:
A: i, v.   **B:** ii, iii.   **C:** iii, v.   **D:** ii, v

(the correct answer is C)

When tackling **exam essays**, remember the following.

Read the question carefully, and try to identify exactly what the examiner is asking for (e.g. is the question limited to innate or adaptive responses, or should you include both? Are details of a single pathway required, or do you need to integrate material from various parts of your course to answer the question fully? If so, do you know all those topics well enough to provide a balanced answer?).

For a one hour essay, spend at least 5 minutes planning at the start—it may seem scary when everyone else appears to have launched straight in, but your essay will be coherent and well-structured, and planning makes sure that you don't forget to include critical points, and that you can balance the material appropriately. Preparation is key here—it really helps if you have already thought out various different essay plans for every conceivable way a question could be asked on each topic, as this saves a lot of time in exams; the pressure is much less if you are confident that you have prepared thoroughly. There is no single correct way to plan an essay—some people make mind maps, others prefer lists, but do make sure that you don't waste time writing full prose (save that for the essay; you can use abbreviations as much as you like in a plan). As you are writing, do keep checking your plan to make sure you include everything you think important.

Avoid waffle—every word needs to count so make sure it's scientific and conveys information quickly, clearly and coherently. Do make sure you use technical terms correctly and spell scientific words carefully. Examiners are not just looking for factual content but evidence that you understand the material and you can demonstrate this by using a clear essay structure (subheadings can really help guide the examiner in your thought processes—check if it's permitted at your institution) and by providing a cogent argument.

Try to include an introduction, the core material and if time, a rounded conclusion.

The **introduction** should contain a *definition* of the key terminology of the question at the start of your answer. You can pick up marks quickly this way and begin the essay in a convincing manner (e.g. 'The activation of naive CD4 expressing helper T lymphocytes expressing a particular T cell antigen receptor which can bind specifically to an MHC-peptide complex presented by a dendritic cell in the lymph node is central to the activation of adaptive immune responses. . . ' sounds rather more scientific than 'Helper T cells are important in activating adaptive immune responses'—a statement that is equally true but much less precise). You can also set the scope of the essay, e.g. 'I shall discuss activation of type 1 interferon responses predominantly, but will touch on other anti-viral effector mechanisms where appropriate. . . '

Paragraphs in the **main body** of the essay should contain:

- Key **concepts**, with details of the immune process (as relevant)
- Specific **named example**(s)
- **Experimental evidence** to support the ideas (even when not specifically asked for in the question). By providing support, you show the examiner that you understand how information was obtained and how strong the evidence is behind the idea—it's a great way of bumping up marks. As you progress through your degree, you will be expected to refer directly to experiments in the primary research literature, so get into the habit of providing experimental evidence early on and it will make it much easier later
- If possible, illustrate with an **annotated diagram**, e.g. draw out the pathway/process (*simply* but clearly—you are being marked on scientific content not artistic merit). Remember that diagrams are only of exam value if they are fully annotated (i.e. have descriptive labels) and **don't take longer to show ideas than it would have taken you to write text describing them**. In most Universities, it is fine to use colour in diagrams, but do check first. The diagrams in this book are intended to be simple and easy to reproduce under exam conditions (though we couldn't use colour because of printing constraints). Don't repeat the same material in diagrams and text, but do introduce each diagram, e.g. 'the protein structure of the T cell antigen receptor (TCR) is shown:' (and remember to use full labels that are clear, legible and informative—so in this case you would identify the alpha and beta chains, plus the associated CD3 chains and its signalling motifs)
- Ensure that you leave sufficient space around your diagrams so the reader can easily see what you are illustrating—don't squeeze them into the margins or wrap text around them
- Comparative tables can also be really helpful to convey factual information rapidly and show the examiner that you can identify key concepts and relate the details to those concepts (e.g. concept: somatic recombination of T cell antigen receptor and B cell antigen receptor lymphocyte genomic DNA; details: the analogous V, J, D gene segments and recombination machinery, i.e. RAG-1 and RAG-2 required to produce rearranged receptors involved in each step), but

make sure you don't rely wholly on such tables, as you will also be marked on the coherency of your discussion

- Round off each paragraph with how the information you have just presented addresses the question

Try to include a **Conclusion** where you can argue for/against (especially if it's a 'Discuss. . .' type essay). You can throw in the odd quirky example here if it didn't fit well into the rest of the essay, but make sure it's relevant. If there are controversies in the field, you can mention them here. Don't waste time repeating things you have already mentioned. You could even highlight what further knowledge is required to fully understand the process (but make sure it's a real gap in knowledge, not simply that you didn't know it!).

Good luck in your exams and do remember that Immunology is a fascinating subject to enjoy—it's not just about passing tests!

Anne C. Cunningham

Brunei
September 2015

Acknowledgements

I would like to thank my son Luke and husband Neil for their encouragement and support. All the members of the 'Abs Fab' training group (Tracey, Nurol, Faye, Mas, Maudena, Surita, Ihsan, Ya Chee, Shirley, David and Ayub. . .) for all the hiking and breakfasts! They have given me the energy to persevere with this rather long 'Friday project'. Many thanks to Jonathan and Martha (OUP) for all their patience, help and support. Finally, I want to thank all my students (past and present) for helping me further appreciate this marvellous and interesting subject!

Abbreviations

ADCC	Antibody dependent cellular cytoxicity
AIDS	Acquired immunodeficiency syndrome
APC	Antigen-presenting cell
AR	Activating receptor
ATP	Adenosine triphosphate
BCR	B cell antigen receptor
C	Complement
CCL	Chemokine (C-C motif) ligand
CCP	Complement control proteins
CCR	Chemokine (C-C motif) receptor
CD	Cluster of differentiation
CpG	Un-methylated cytidine-phosphate-guanosine dinucleotides
CR	Complement receptor
CRP	C reactive protein
CSF	Colony stimulating factors
CTL	Cytotoxic T lymphocyte
CXCL	Chemokine (C-X-C motif) ligand
CXCR	Chemokine (C-X-C motif) receptor
CX3L	Chemokine (C-X3-C motif) ligand
CX3R	Chemokine (C-X3-C motif) receptor
DAG	Diacylglycerol
DAF	Decay accelerating factor
DAMP	Damage-associated molecular patterns
DC	Dendritic cell
ds	Double stranded
ER	Endoplasmic reticulum
GALT	Gut associated lymphoid tissue
γC	Common gamma chain
GC	Germinal Centre
HIV	Human immunodeficiency virus
HLA	Human leukocyte antigens
HSCT	Haematopoietic stem cell transplantation
IBD	Inflammatory bowel disease
IFN	Interferons
Ig	Immunoglobulin
IL	Interleukin
IP3	Inositol 1,4,5 triphosphate
IR	Inhibitory receptor
IRF	Interferon regulatory factor
ISG	Interferon stimulated genes

Abbreviations

ITAM	Immuno-receptor tyrosine-based activation motif
LAMP	Lysosome-associated membrane proteins
LCA	Leucocyte common antigen
LPS	Lipopolysaccharide
LRR	Leucine rich repeats
MASP	MBL associated serine proteases
MBL	Mannan binding lectin
MCP	Membrane cofactor protein
MHC	Major Histocompatibility Complex
MR	Mannose receptor
NCRs	Natural cytotoxicity receptors
NETs	Neutrophil extracellular traps
NFAT	Nuclear factor of activated T cells
NK	Natural killer cells
NKL	Natural killer cell ligand
NLR	Nod-like receptors
NOD	nuclear oligomerization domains
PALS	Periarteriolar lymphoid sheaths
PAMP	Pathogen-associated molecular patterns
PBMC	Peripheral blood mononuclear cells
PBR	Peptide Binding Region
PLC	Phospholipase C
PMN	Polymorphonuclear cells
PRR	Pattern recognition receptor
PTX3	Pentraxin 3
RAG	Recombination activating gene
RCA	Regulators of complement activation
RIG	Retinoic acid inducible gene
RLR	RIG-like receptors
RNS	Reactive nitrogen species
ROS	Reactive oxygen species
SAP	Serum amyloid component
SP-A	Surfactant protein A
TAP	Transporter associated with Antigen Processing
TCR	T cell antigen receptor
Th	T helper
SCID	Severe combined immunodeficiency
ss	single stranded
TLR	Toll-like receptor
TNFα	Tumour necrosis factor alpha
VJDC	Variable Joining Diversity Constant gene segments
WBC	White blood cells
WHO	World Health Organization
XCL	Chemokine (C motif) ligand
XCR	Chemokine (C motif) receptor

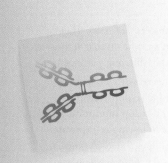

1 Introduction to Immune Responses, Cells, Mediators, and Structures

The immune system is a whole body system—but it can be a struggle to see the 'bigger picture' and make connections between different elements of the immune system and the many responses it mediates. The other challenge is in understanding the language used to describe immune responses. Please consult the glossary terms (defined in the Glossary) which are highlighted in the text.

This revision guide is designed to support your learning of immunology and may not be written in exactly the same way you have been taught on your course. It aims to help you understand how different elements of the immune system can recognize (Chapter 2: introduces the receptors, what they bind to and the subsequent responses mediated) and destroy (Chapter 3: introduces the key effector mechanisms that lead to destruction) things that are dangerous, i.e pathogens and tumour cells. This first chapter introduces the key concepts plus the structures, cells and mediators of the immune response. You will find more details on nomenclature at the end of this chapter.

Key concepts in immunity

- There are two integrated systems (**innate immunity** and **adaptive immunity**) which work together to eradicate **pathogens** and limit the development of **tumours**.

continued

- Innate responses are present in all organisms (plants, insects, animals). They don't change following repeated exposure and are 'non-specific' in that activation by one pathogen will lead to an increased killing of other different pathogens.
- Adaptive immune responses are only present in organisms with a backbone (vertebrates) and a jaw. You can make a specific immune response against absolutely anything (*specificity* and *diversity*). You also develop immunological *memory*, so will make a much faster *escalating response* following re-exposure.
- All white blood cells (**leukocytes**) are 'innate cells' with the exception of **lymphocytes**, which are the ONLY cells responsible for making adaptive immune responses.
- The key difference between the innate and adaptive immune responses is the way they recognize pathogens (different types of receptors).
- Immune responses are compartmentalized. They are induced and resolved in tissues, but depend on cellular activation in draining **lymph nodes**.
- The production and activation of leukocytes are controlled by mediators called **cytokines**.
- The immune system has to cover the whole body and leukocytes are mobile. Their movement is controlled by mediators called **chemokines**.

1.1 PURPOSE AND OVERVIEW OF THE IMMUNE SYSTEM

The immune system recognizes and destroys things that are DANGEROUS. These are agents or conditions that cause harm to the body. The danger signals can come from outside the body (exogenous, e.g. viral RNA, bacterial cell walls) or from damaged cells (endogenous, e.g. extracellular ATP, heat shock proteins). They lead to the generation of alarm signals which alert and activate immune responses. In a well-functioning immune system, the signals from the tissues instruct the quantity and the quality of the specific immune responses required to eradicate any danger that is present.

Key features of the immune system

- The immune system needs to be focused toward our barriers with the external environment. These include the mucosa (lungs, gastrointestinal tract, and genitourinary system) and the skin.
- Infectious agents enter via our external surfaces. The majority of infectious diseases affect the lung (respiratory diseases), gastrointestinal tract (diarrhoea caused by infectious gastroenteritis or food poisoning), or gain entry through the skin (diseases carried by biting insects, e.g. malaria).
- Pathogens generally first bind body cells to gain entry, and then cause damage in tissue which leads to the activation of signals and the generation of **inflammation**.
- Responses in tissue are detected by cells draining to the **lymph nodes**.

- Recognition is mediated by receptors.
- Receptor binding leads to activation of immune response genes.
- Adaptive immune responses are generated in lymph nodes.
- Adaptive immune responses are mediated by **lymphocytes** (T and B cells).

Barriers

- Physical barriers are the first line of defence against pathogens. They consist of the mucosa and skin.
- Epithelial cells line the interface between the body and the external environment. They form good barriers because of their tight junctions.
- These barriers co-ordinate a range of non-specific and specific defences. For example,
  - Ciliated epithelial cells lining the airways sweep inhaled agents upwards (mucociliary escalator) and out of the lung.
  - Goblet cells at mucosal surfaces secrete mucus which contains a complex mixture of glycoproteins/enzymes (e.g. lysozyme) which can bind to/digest bacterial cell walls.
  - Surfactant-producing cells (in the lung and gastrointestinal tract) secrete molecules (e.g. surfactant protein A and D) which bind directly to pathogen cell walls to facilitate their destruction by macrophages.
  - Mucosal epithelial cells express a poly-Ig receptor which binds to dimeric IgA and enables its trans-epithelial transport and the formation of secretory IgA which blocks the binding of pathogen to the mucosal surfaces. (See Chapter 3, section 3.2, Antibodies as effector molecules.)

Looking for extra marks?

Humans make their own 'antibiotics'—and synthesize a range of anti-microbial peptides including α and β **defensins**. These highly conserved molecules produced by **neutrophils** and epithelial cells, can insert into pathogen cell walls and disturb their membranes leading to pore formation.

1.2 INFLAMMATION

Inflammation is a physiological response to injury and is characterized by five cardinal signs (heat, pain, redness, swelling, loss of function). Its purpose is to focus immune responses where they are needed. It leads to the accumulation of leukocytes (e.g. **neutrophils**), and mediators (e.g. **acute phase proteins**) from the blood into the tissue (Figure 1.1). Accumulated cells and mediators will recognize and/or destroy pathogens or contribute to the repair process. In healthy individuals with a normal immune system, the infection will be resolved and the tissue should be functionally restored.

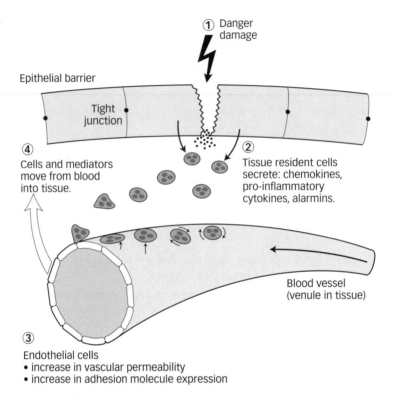

Figure 1.1 Overview of the inflammatory immune response which focuses responses where they are needed. Epithelial barriers line all our external environment (skin, mucosa) and form tight junctions. If there is injury or infection (1), this barrier can be breached enabling microbes to gain entry to underlying tissue. Tissue resident cells respond by secreting mediators which attract and activate leukocytes (2). This happens because pro-inflammatory mediators induce changes in the endothelial cells of blood vessels (3) so they become 'stickier' and 'leakier'. This enables leukocytes to adhere to the endothelial cells and ultimately migrate from the blood vessel into the tissue (4) where they accumulate at the focus of infection or injury.

Acute local inflammation

These are local changes that take place in damaged tissue. They can be induced by a wide range of agents including:

- Infection by pathogens (e.g. viruses, bacteria, fungi, parasites).
- Release of bacterial toxins.
- Trauma/injury.
- Ultraviolet or other harmful radiation.
- Burns or frostbite.
- Irritant/corrosive chemicals (e.g. acids, alkalis, oxidizing agents).

- Tissue necrosis which results from the toxic build-up of dead cells and cellular debris in affected tissue.
- Hypersensitivity reactions (to microbes, plants or other materials).

Key features of acute local inflammation

- Rapid onset and short duration.
- Tissue resident cells which have been damaged (e.g. by the agents listed above) or have received danger (or alarm) signals release **chemokines** (*chemo*tactic cyto*kines*) which function to recruit leukocytes into the tissue. They can also release pro-inflammatory mediators, e.g. tumour necrosis factor alpha (**TNFα**) and **interferon gamma** which modify blood vessel endothelial cells (Figure 1.1).
- This leads to changes in blood vessels, i.e an increase in vascular permeability and **adhesion molecule** expression.
- Circulating leukocytes adhere to blood vessel endothelial cells—first rolling, then tightly adhering before transmigrating into the tissue.
- This leads to the accumulation of leukocytes within tissues:
  - **Neutrophils** (the most common white blood cell) arrive first (within minutes) and destroy pathogens by **phagocytosis**.
  - **Monocytes** differentiate into **macrophages** where they destroy pathogens by phagocytosis but also contribute to the inflammatory cascade by producing pro-inflammatory **cytokines**.
- Pro-inflammatory cytokines, e.g. **TNFα**, **interleukin 1 beta** (**IL-1β**) and IL-6, promote the inflammatory cascade and also increase in the circulation to stimulate systemic inflammation.

Revision Tip

Remember, local inflammation focuses effective responses at the site of infection or damage. It is characterized by:

- *vascular changes*
  - vasodilation
  - increase in vascular permeability and exudation of plasma proteins
- *cellular events*
  - increased adhesion and transmigration of leukocytes leading to the recruitment of inflammatory cells into the tissue.
- *activation*
  - pro-inflammatory cytokine secretion and activation of inflammatory cells (leukocytes)

Inflammation

1. **What can cause the vascular changes observed in blood vessels in inflamed tissue?**
- Cytokines, e.g. TNFα, IL-1β, IL-6 (which also play a role in systemic inflammation) and many others which act locally, e.g. interferon gamma (IFNγ).
- Lipid mediators (metabolites of arachadonic acid including thromboxane, prostaglandins, leukotrienes and platelet activating factor).
- Kallikrein-kinin system (e.g. bradykinin).
- Clotting system (e.g. thrombin, fibrin).
- Fibrinolytic system (e.g. plasmin).
- Complement proteins (e.g. C3a, C4a and C5a).
- Mast cell products (including TNFα, lipid mediators, histamine and many more).

2. **How do leukocytes migrate into tissue?**
- Normally leukocytes will travel at the speed of blood flow in the centre of vessels.
- Inflammation causes vasodilation which causes the slowing down of blood flow in affected tissue.
- Pro-inflammatory cytokines cause endothelial cells to upregulate **adhesion molecule** expression. For example, **TNFα** causes the surface expression of pre-formed p-**selectin** from 'Weibel-Palade' bodies in endothelial cells. **TNFα** also causes upregulation of e-**selectin** and members of the Ig Superfamily **adhesion molecules** (e.g. ICAM-1, ICAM-2, ICAM-3, VCAM-1) on the surface of endothelial cells.
- Leukocytes first roll along the blood vessel wall by making and breaking low affinity interactions between their surface expressed glycoproteins (e.g. sialyl-lewis^x) and **selectins** on endothelial cells (see rolling leukocytes in Figure 1.1).
- Leukocyte **integrins** then bind to ICAMs on endothelial cells causing them to stop. Chemokines bound to the surface of endothelial cells can activate the leukocytes to upregulate the affinity of their integrins so they bind tightly to the blood vessel wall (see flattened leukocyte in Figure 1.1).
- The leukocyte then squeezes between two adjacent endothelial cells in a process known as extravasation or diapedesis.
- The directional movement of leukocytes is mediated by **chemokines**, so they accumulate at the sites of tissue injury or infection.

Revision tip

Adhesion molecules are like molecular 'Velcro'. The blood vessel walls upregulate the 'loops' during inflammation and since leukocytes express the 'hooks' they will stick to blood vessel walls in inflamed tissue. Once stuck, they will follow the chemotactic signals and crawl into the tissue.

Acute systemic inflammation

- Local inflammation leads to the up-regulation of three key pro-inflammatory cytokines (**TNFα**, **IL-1**, IL-6) which can have effects on other parts of the body.

- They induce fever (via the hypothalamus, the temperature-regulating centre found at the base of the brain) and are therefore sometimes referred to as 'endogenous pyrogens'.
- They promote the production of more leukocytes in the **bone marrow** (by induction of 'colony stimulating factors').
- They stimulate the acute phase response (Figure 1.2).
- Acute phase proteins (particularly C-reactive protein CRP) are useful indicators of systemic inflammation. They are produced by hepatocytes (in the liver) and their serum concentrations increase many fold (Table 1.1).
- This group of serum proteins are rapidly (12–24h) produced in the liver in response to an increase in systemic concentrations of these pro-inflammatory cytokines (**TNFα, IL-1**, IL-6). They play a key role in assisting recognition and destruction of pathogens, plus contribute to the repair process.

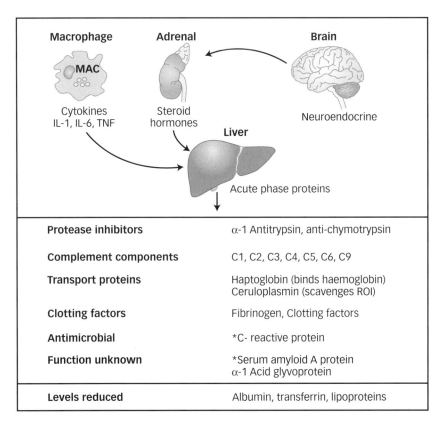

Protease inhibitors	α-1 Antitrypsin, anti-chymotrypsin
Complement components	C1, C2, C3, C4, C5, C6, C9
Transport proteins	Haptoglobin (binds haemoglobin) Ceruloplasmin (scavenges ROI)
Clotting factors	Fibrinogen, Clotting factors
Antimicrobial	*C- reactive protein
Function unknown	*Serum amyloid A protein α-1 Acid glyvoprotein
Levels reduced	Albumin, transferrin, lipoproteins

Figure 1.2 An illustration of how locally produced pro-inflammatory cytokines enter the circulation and induce a systemic response, in particular upregulating the production of acute phase proteins by the liver.

Source: Infection and Immunity, Fourth edition by John Playfair and Gregory Bancroft (2013). By permission of Oxford University Press. © John Playfair and Gregory Bancroft.

Inflammation

Acute phase protein	Serum concentration
C reactive protein (CRP)	68–8200 mg/L
alpha acid glycoprotein	550–1400 mg/L
alpha-1-antitrypsin	0.78–2 g/L
ceruplasmin	1.8–4.5 g/L
haptoglobin	350–1640 mg/L

Table 1.1 Examples of acute phase proteins (typical adult values).

> ## Revision Tip
>
> Remember CRP is a useful but non-specific indicator of acute systemic inflammation. It can be raised during infection, but also in cancer. It is a common biomedical laboratory test requested in hospital pathology laboratories to help clinicians determine the extent of systemic inflammation in patients. It cannot be used to determine the cause of inflammation.

Chronic inflammation

- Chronic inflammation results if acute inflammation fails to remove an 'insult' which has caused damage.
- This results from the *persistence* of the factors which stimulated inflammation. It leads to excessive repair and the development of tissue remodelling, including fibrosis. (See Table 1.2 for examples of chronic inflammatory diseases.)
- Fibrosis is defined as a 'loss of structure, deposition of extracellular matrix and increase in inflammatory cells'.
- Interestingly the most pro-inflammatory cells and mediators are also the most fibrogenic, including:
  - Mast cells
  - Thrombin
  - Fibrinogen peptides
- A granuloma is an ancient tissue response which walls off any agent that cannot be removed. They are characterized by a central area of activated macrophages (which may be fused to form multi-nucleated 'giant cells'), and they are commonly surrounded by leukocytes (e.g. eosinophils, T lymphocytes). They may calcify over time. Pathologists often describe the macrophages in granulomas as 'epithelioid' in appearance.

Site	Disease
Gut	Inflammatory bowel disease (IBD), e.g. Crohn's disease, ulcerative colitis
Pancreas	Diabetes Mellitus
Synovium	Rheumatoid Arthritis
Thyroid	Grave's disease, Hashimoto's thyroiditis
Lung	Asthma

Table 1.2 Examples of chronic inflammatory diseases.

> ## Key features of chronic inflammation
>
> - The accumulation and activation of macrophages.
> - Release of pro-inflammatory cytokines.
> - Fibroblast proliferation and collagen deposition.
> - Fibrosis/granuloma formation.

Revision Tip

A pearl is caused by a foreign body in a shellfish (mollusc) which calcifies over time due to the build-up of calcium carbonate. A granuloma is a focus of inflammatory cells which may also calcify as a result of tissue remodelling. Imagine the immune system is simply 'walling up' something it cannot remove in order to contain it.

1.3 INNATE IMMUNITY

- Innate or 'inborn' responses are described as 'non-specific'. It is more accurate to consider them as cross reactive. For example an innate receptor may not be able to discriminate between specific pathogens, but be activated by all gram-negative bacteria expressing lipopolysaccharide (**LPS**).
- Innate responses are present in all multicellular organisms. They are highly conserved, so the same genes (e.g. **Toll pathway**) found in a fruit fly or a nematode worm are responsible for innate responses in humans (e.g. **Toll-like receptor, TLR**). Interestingly, *all* eukaryotic organisms use the **NF-κβ** signal transduction pathway to activate immune response genes following infection.
- All white blood cells are innate cells, with the exception of **lymphocytes**.
- All innate receptors are 'biased' to things that are dangerous—structures associated with pathogens or released by damaged cells.
- Danger (or alarm) signals from damaged or stressed cells can also activate innate immune responses.
- Danger signals fall into two categories (Table 1.3):
  - intracellular components found outside of the cell—indicating necrotic or inflammatory cell death (**pyroptosis**)
  - elements of pathogens which are structurally different from mammalian cells (e.g. in the organization of sugars, nucleic acids, etc.)

Exogenous	Endogenous
Lipopolysaccharide	Extracellular ATP
Peptidoglycan	Hypotonic stress
Flagella	Uric acid crystals
Double-stranded RNA	Heat shock proteins

Table 1.3 Some 'danger' signals which initiate innate immune responses

- Successful pathogens evade immune responses by evolving mechanisms to avoid recognition or destruction or actively suppress immune responses.
- More information on how the innate immune system recognizes (Chapter 2) and destroys (Chapter 3) pathogens is provided in later chapters.

Key features of innate immune responses

- Rapid (minutes).
- Cross reactive (non-specific).
- Does not change following repeated exposure.
- Many different types of receptors that recognize 'dangerous molecules' (pathogen-associated molecular patterns **PAMPs** or damage-associated molecular patterns **DAMPs**).
- Generally recognize carbohydrates and lipids.
- Once activated, innate effector mechanism can destroy all pathogens more effectively (i.e. they are non-specific).
- Stimulate specific immune responses (adaptive immunity).

Revision Tip

Remember, a receptor that can bind to a carbohydrate with high affinity is called a lectin.

1.4 ADAPTIVE IMMUNITY

Adaptive immune responses are only present in organisms with a backbone (vertebrates) and a jaw. They exist in fish, reptiles, birds and mammals. The only cell types responsible for mediating adaptive immune responses are **lymphocytes**.

Key features of adaptive immune responses

- Only lymphocytes (T and B cells).
- Adaptive immune responses are *diverse*, *specific* and characterized by *memory*, which leads to an *escalating response* upon re-exposure.
- Lymphocytes are clonal (i.e one cell will divide to produce many identical daughter cells).
- Lymphocytes express rearranged receptors (**T cell antigen receptor, TCR** and **B cell antigen receptor, BCR**) which are highly variable.
- They generally recognize protein conformation (BCR)/peptides (TCR).
- Once activated, adaptive effector responses are specific to the stimulus (unlike innate immune responses).

- Adaptive receptors are randomly rearranged so are not 'biased' to infectious agents (like innate receptors). We all generate a unique 'repertoire' of lymphocyte receptors (TCR and BCR) to enable us to fight infection.
- Adaptive immune responses are necessary to specifically eradicate pathogens.
- More information is provided in later chapters on how the adaptive immune system recognizes (Chapter 2) and destroys (Chapter 3) pathogens.

Revision Tip

Patients who do not have lymphocytes cannot fight infection and have a severe combined immunodeficiency (SCID). They experience repeated bacterial infections, fail to thrive and will die in early childhood unless they receive a bone marrow transplant. This illustrates that however good innate immune responses are, they are not enough to eradicate pathogens alone.

Primary immune response

- A lymphocyte that has never been activated is referred to as 'naive'.
- Naive T lymphocytes (or T cells) generally travel around the blood and transit through secondary lymphoid organs (e.g. lymph nodes and **spleen**).
- Naive B lymphocytes (or B cells) generally reside in B cell areas of lymph nodes.
- Only specialized **antigen-presenting cells** (APC i.e dendritic cells) can activate naive T cells and activate adaptive immune responses.
- If a lymphocyte can bind specifically to an **antigen** (e.g. strain A of a pathogen, see Figure 1.3) which has been carried by an APC to a secondary lymphoid organ then it is selected for activation.
- T cell activation involves a number of steps which will instruct the kind of response generated (see Chapter 2 for more detail):
  - Specific recognition of an 'antigen'
  - Costimulation
  - Cytokine signal
- The costimulatory and cytokine signals are upregulated by inflammation/innate immune responses. They direct the quality and quantity of the specifc adaptive immune response and reflect the type of infection in the tissue.
- Following activation, the lymphocyte (B or T) which is specific (i.e it bears a useful receptor that can bind to a particular antigen, e.g. strain A of a pathogen, see Figure 1.3) proliferates to create many identical daughter cells (e.g. 10^2–10^3) which further differentiate to mediate the specific immune response to recognize and destroy that pathogen (strain A, see Figure 1.3).
- Activated helper T cells then help B cells to make **antibodies** (anti-strain A antibodies, see Figure 1.3) in secondary lymphoid organs.

Adaptive immunity

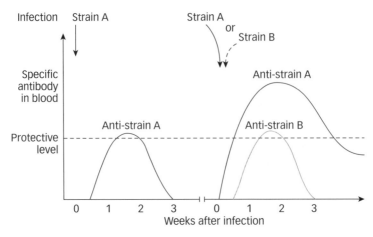

Figure 1.3 The first time the body is exposed to a pathogen (e.g. strain A) a primary immune response is mediated (anti-strain A) which will control infection in 1–2 weeks. A second exposure will lead to a much more rapid (2–3 days) and larger secondary immune response, illustrated by the higher levels of anti-strain A antibodies. This is specific because if the body is also exposed to a different pathogen (e.g. strain B) at the same time, then a slower primary immune response (anti-strain B) is made. This illustrates the fundamental properties of the adaptive immune response, i.e. specificity (A is different to B), diversity (responses can be made to A and B, etc.), escalating responses (the second exposure to strain A leads to the faster and larger secondary immune response) and immunological memory (strain A was remembered).

Source: *Infection and Immunity*, Fourth Edition by John Playfair and Gregory Bancroft (2013). By permission of Oxford University Press. © John Playfair and Gregory Bancroft.

- Specific differentiated effector cells and antibodies home back to the tissue and resolve the infection.
- **Primary immune responses** take time (7–10 days; cellular activation, proliferation, differentiation) and are characterized by increases in specific **IgM** (serum) (Figure 1.3).
- At the end of the immune response, the majority of effector cells (90–95%) will be removed (activation induced cell death) and a population of **memory cells** (T and B lymphocytes) will remain.
- Some memory T cells continue to recirculate around the whole body, and are referred to as 'central memory' T cells (T_{CM}). They can be found in secondary lymphoid organs and blood. Effector memory T cells (T_{EM}) recirculate between the tissue where the original infection started and its draining lymph node (but not the blood). Another population of memory cells has been found to stay in the tissue (tissue resident memory T cells T_{RM}), particularly the skin and mucosal surfaces (lung, gastrointestinal tract, vagina) but are not found in secondary lymphoid organs or blood.

Secondary immune responses

- Following initial exposure the adaptive immune system is 'sensitized' and can respond more quickly following re-exposure to the same agent. This is called immunological memory.
- Lymphocytes (T and B) which have been previously activated can differentiate into populations of memory cells.
- Memory T cells are easier to activate than naive T cells, and because there are more of them surveying the likely site of infection, they can respond much more rapidly if re-exposed to the same pathogen (e.g. strain A, Figure 1.3).
- Memory B cells will reside in the lymph nodes which drain the previously infected tissue.
- **Secondary immune responses** are rapid (2–3 days) and high levels of specific **IgG** may be seen in the serum (Figure 1.3).
- Vaccination is a very effective public health measure which relies on the principles of adaptive immunity. The vaccine induces a primary immune response, so that when we are later exposed to the vaccine-specific infectious agent, we make a rapid secondary immune response which (ideally) destroys the pathogen and we are protected from disease (Figure 1.4, Table 1.4).

Adaptive immunity

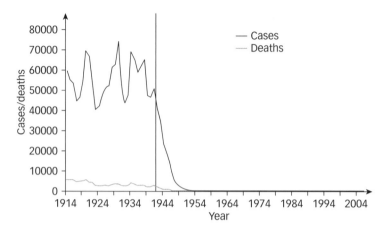

Figure 1.4 Diptheria cases and deaths in England and Wales (1914–2004). The vaccine was introduced in 1942.

© Crown Copyright (Health Protection Agency, now Public Health England)

Disease (pathogen)	Vaccine
Anthrax (*Bacillus anthracis*)	Inactivated vaccine (suspension of sterile filtrate from *B. anthracis* cultures)
Cholera (*Vibrio Cholerae*)	Killed *V. cholerae* whole-cell (WC) vaccine with recombinant B subunit of cholera toxin (rCTB)
Diptheria (*Corynebacterium diphtheria*)	Cell-free purified toxin extracted from *C. diphtheriae* treated with formaldehyde to produce a toxoid vaccine
Hepatitis A (Hepatitis A virus)	Purified inactivated virus (monovalent) or combined with Hep B (purified recombinant hepatitis B surface antigen)
Hepatitis B (Hepatitis B virus)	Purified recombinant hepatitis B surface antigen
Influenza (Influenza virus, generally type A or B)	Combinations of inactivated subunit vaccines (prepared using virus strains according to WHO recommendations). Generally trivalent (i.e containing the subunits from three prevalent viral strains) or quadrivalent (extracts from four strains included)
Measles (morbillivirus)	Live, attenuated strain of measles virus (in combination with mumps and rubella vaccine = MMR)
Mumps (paramyxovirus)	Live, attenuated strain of measles virus (in combination with measles and rubella vaccine = MMR)
Pneumococcal (*Streptococcus pneumoniae*)	Purified capsular polysaccharide (from multiple strains)
Polio (poliovirus serotypes 1, 2 and 3)	Inactivated polio vaccine (IPV) contains 3 strains (serotypes 1,2,3) and given in combination with diphtheria (D)/tetanus (T)/acellular pertussis (aP)/*Haemophilus influenzae* type b (Hib) vaccine (e.g. DTaP/IPV/Hib or DTaP/IPV or Td/IPV) Live attenuated vaccine (OPV) may be used for outbreak control
Rabies (lyssaviruses)	Inactivated virus
Rotavirus (rotavirus)	Live attenuated virus strain

Rubella (togavirus)	Live, attenuated strain of rubella virus (given in combination with measles and mumps vaccine = MMR)
Tetanus (*Clostridium tetani*)	Cell-free purified toxin extracted from a strain of *C. tetani* treated with formaldehyde to produce a toxoid vaccine
Typhoid (*Salmonella enterica* serotype *typhi* or *paratyphi*)	Purified Vi capsular polysaccharide from *S. typhi* An oral live attenuated strain of *S. typhi* and killed whole cell inactivated *S. typhi* vaccine exist
Whooping Cough (*Bordetella pertussis*)	Acellular vaccines from highly purified components of the *B.pertussis* (aP) given in combination with diphtheria (D)/tetanus (T)/polio (P)/*Haemophilus influenza* type b (Hib) e.g. DTaP/IPV/Hib
Yellow fever (flavivirus)	Live attenuated virus strain

Table 1.4 Examples of vaccine preventable disease

Source the 'Green Book': Immunization against infectious disease, Public Health England https://www.gov.uk/government/collections/immunisation-against-infectious-disease-the-green-book#part-2-the-diseases-vaccinations-and-vaccines

1.5 STRUCTURE, CELLS AND MEDIATORS OF THE IMMUNE SYSTEM

You can be infected by many different agents in every part of your body. The structures, cells and mediators of the immune system are widely distributed (Figure 1.5).

- All leukocytes are formed in the bone marrow.
- Inflammation is the body's response to danger in tissue. The main function is to recruit inflammatory cells and mediators from the blood into the tissue.
- Inflammation also promotes the 'capture' of infectious agents in the tissue by the transit of specialized 'antigen-presenting cells' to secondary lymphoid organs.
- Antigen-presenting cells play a key role in activating T lymphocytes and adaptive immune responses.
- Adaptive immune responses are generated in organized lymphoid tissue (secondary lymphoid organs) and the effector cells then traffic back to the tissue.

Structures—primary lymphoid organs

These are sites of leukocyte production and/or lymphocyte maturation. There are two primary lymphoid organs—the bone marrow and thymus. The process of lymphocyte maturation involves the formation of the **T cell antigen receptor (TCR)** and the **B cell antigen receptor (BCR)**. More information on lymphocyte receptors is provided in Chapter 2.

1. Bone marrow

- Found in the central cavities of axial and long bones.
- Major haematopoietic organ and the primary site of haematopoiesis (formation of red blood cells, all leukocytes and platelets).

Structure, cells and mediators of the immune system

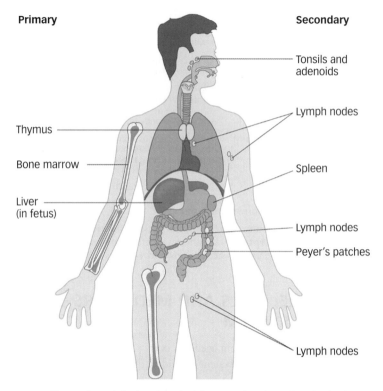

Figure 1.5 An illustration of the key lymphoid organs distributed in the body.

Source: Infection and Immunity, Fourth Edition by John Playfair and Gregory Bancroft (2013). By permission of Oxford University Press. © John Playfair and Gregory Bancroft.

- Specialized microenvironment which contains stem cells and growth factors (including colony-stimulating factors CSFs).
- Pluripotent stem cells self-renew and can give rise to all haematopoietic cells (erythrocytes, granulocytes, monocytes, lymphocytes, platelets, see Figure 1.8).
- They are rapidly growing cells so any agents that target dividing cells (radioactivity, cytotoxic drugs) will interfere with bone marrow function and the production of red and white blood cells.

What else does the bone marrow do?
- The bone marrow is also the site of B lymphocyte development and maturation.
- Pre-B cells do not express any antigen receptor (**BCR**) until they have gone through the random process of receptor rearrangement, which leads to receptor diversity (Chapter 2).
- Some of the newly generated BCR will be auto-reactive and therefore potentially dangerous.
- Those BCR which can bind to self antigens with high affinity are deleted by apoptosis. This is called *negative selection*.

- Other BCR do not bind to self, and continue to differentiate into mature B cells which are positively selected into the circulation and secondary lymphoid organs.
- The B cell receptor complex consists of membrane-bound immunoglobulin M (IgM), complexed with two associated immunoglobulin chains (Igα or CD79a and Igβ or CD79b).
- It has been estimated that you generate over 10^{11} different kinds of B cells based on BCR variability.

Revision Tip

Questions commonly ask about the effects of agents that interfere with bone marrow function. The consequence will be a reduction in the full blood count and immunosuppression. Patients will be at increased risk of infections.

Looking for extra marks?

All bone-marrow-derived cells can be identified by the surface marker CD45. It is also known as the Leucocyte Common Antigen (LCA). It is the major tyrosine phosphatase found in leukocyte plasma membranes. It plays a key role in the signalling pathways required for the activation of T and B lymphocytes. Stem cells can be identified by the expression of the surface glycoprotein, CD34.

2. Thymus

- Lobed, capsulated organ found in the upper thorax.
- It is very active before birth and during childhood, peaks in size at puberty and then dwindles with age.
- Unique environment to promote the development and maturation of T lymphocytes.
- Immature 'thymocytes' traffic from the bone marrow to the cortex where they begin to express functional T cell antigen receptors (**TCR**) following the random rearrangement of their TCR alpha and beta chains (Chapter 2).
- A small proportion of lymphocytes (<10%) also express TCR with rearranged gamma and delta chains.
- Newly formed TCR interact with cortical epithelial cells. This is to select those randomly generated TCR which can bind to self-molecules (**MHC**/peptide complexes). Any TCR which don't bind to 'self' (MHC/peptide complexes) are useless and die by neglect. This is how your T cells become restricted to 'self' (or 'MHC-restricted'). TCR which can bind to self-molecules (MHC/peptide complexes) on cortical epithelial cells with a *low affinity* are *positively selected* to grow (Figure 1.6).
- The maturing T lymphocytes move deeper into the thymic medulla where they interact with thymic epithelial cells, dendritic cells and macrophages. Those TCR which bind with very high affinity to self-molecules (MHC/peptide complexes) are potentially dangerous and are deleted by apoptosis.

Structure, cells and mediators of the immune system

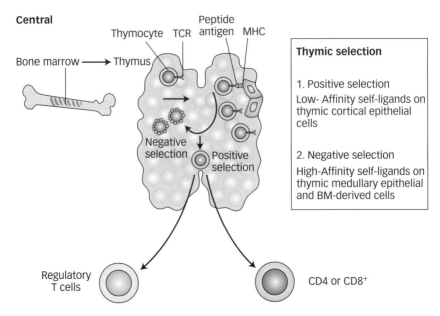

Thymic selection

1. Positive selection
Low- Affinity self-ligands on thymic cortical epithelial cells

2. Negative selection
High-Affinity self-ligands on thymic medullary epithelial and BM-derived cells

Figure 1.6 Illustration of the thymus and the role it plays in the positive and negative selection of T lymphocytes. T cells with an intermediate affinity for self MHC/self-peptide survive the selection process and exit the thymus to join the circulation to mature as **naive lymphocytes** CD4 or CD8. T cells with the highest affinity for self MHC/self-peptide complexes in the thymus that survive negative selection (i.e. deletion) are programmed to be regulatory T cells (Tregs) and specifically switch immune responses off.

Source: P.K. Gregerson and T. W. Behrens 2006, 'Genetics of autoimmune diseases— disorders of immune homeostasis', in *Nature Reviews Genetics*, **7**, 917–228. Reprinted by permission from Macmillan Publishers Ltd: *Nature Reviews Genetics*, copyright 2006.

- This process is referred to as *negative selection* (Figure 1.6). It leads to the destruction of potentially auto-reactive T lymphocytes in the thymus and is very important in limiting autoimmunity. The majority of immature thymocytes with their newly rearranged TCR are deleted at this stage (Chapter 4).
- **Central tolerance** is the consequence of negative selection (i.e deletion) of T lymphocytes which can bind to self-molecules (i.e MHC/self peptide) in the thymus with *high affinity*.
- T cells with a low affinity for self-molecules (MHC/peptide complexes) survive negative selection and leave the thymus to enter the peripheral T cell pool as 'recent thymic emigrants'.
- There is evidence that the development of mature naive T cells takes place soon after they leave the thymus.
- It has been estimated that you have over 10^{16}–10^{18} different kinds of T cells based on variability in TCR alpha and beta chain structure. This is the basis for your highly diverse adaptive immune system.

Revision Tip

Removal of the thymus at birth causes a profound immunosuppression and causes a failure in the development of adaptive immune responses. However removal during adulthood does not seem to be harmful.

Structures—Secondary lymphoid organs

- These function to promote adaptive immune responses.
- They are optimally designed to capture antigen from tissues, concentrate them and present to T and B lymphocytes.
- You will have relatively few specific lymphocyte receptors (BCR or TCR) for any particular pathogen.
- This compartmentalization enables you to concentrate any potential pathogens and increase the chance of you activating lymphocytes with useful receptors that can recognize (and ultimately) destroy the invader.
- Optimal conditions for lymphocyte activation exist within these specialized structures.

Key features

- Possess an arterial blood supply. Vessels are lined with specialized endothelial cells ('**high endothelial venules**' **HEV**) which facilitate the entrance of T lymphocytes. This is the gateway.
- Have a mechanism for antigen entry. This leads to the capture and concentration of pathogens.
- Contain organized T and B cell areas, macrophages and dendritic cells.
- Ideal microenvironment for the activation of T and B cells and the generation of adaptive immune responses.
- Possess efferent lymphatics and an exiting venous blood supply.

1. Lymph nodes
- It is estimated that you have over 500 lymph nodes in your body which are linked by lymphatic vessels to each other.
- They function to capture material (including pathogens) in all tissues, concentrate it and bring it into close contact with T and B cells.
- If any of these lymphocytes have specific receptors (TCR, BCR) for any part of the pathogen, they are activated and an adaptive immune response is generated which results in the proliferation and clonal expansion of these useful receptor-bearing lymphocytes. This ultimately leads to the specific recognition and destruction of invading pathogens.
- Inflammation and infection lead to a massive increase in the size of your lymph nodes. You can feel these easily in your head and neck when you are ill/experiencing 'flu-like' symptoms.

Structure, cells and mediators of the immune system

What is the structure of lymph nodes?
- See Figure 1.7
- Capsulated lobular structures found along lymphatic vessels.
- 'Lymphatic fluid' enters via the afferent lymphatic vessels.
- Contain a reticular meshwork of fibroblasts which frames the three dimensional structure and support clusters of macrophages, dendritic cells and other leukocytes.
- Blood vessels are suspended in this by collagenous cords which are surrounded by fibroblastic reticular cells and lymphocytes.
- Possess a cortex, paracortex (deep cortex) and medulla.
- B cells are found in spherical follicles in the superficial cortex.
- T cells enter the lymph node via specialized blood vessels and travel through the paracortex where they interact with dendritic cells.

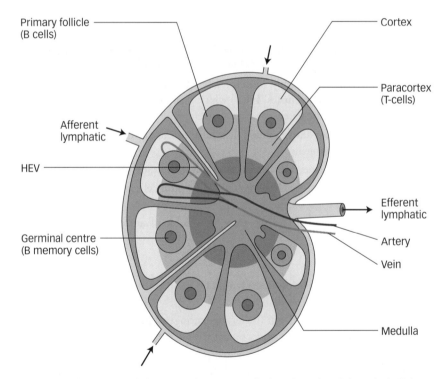

Figure 1.7 Illustration of the general structure of a lymph node. High endothelial venules (HEV) possess specialized adhesion molecules which enable T lymphocytes to bind to them and enter. Pathogens are brought from the tissue via the afferent lymphatics (marked with inward arrows), generally by antigen-presenting cells (e.g. dendritic cells).

Source: *Infection and Immunity*, Fourth Edition by John Playfair and Gregory Bancroft (2013). By permission of Oxford University Press. © John Playfair and Gregory Bancroft.

- A T cell will normally exit the lymph node after about 18h via the efferent lymphatic and eventually join the blood supply at the thoracic duct.
- If a T cell is activated in the paracortex (Chapter 2), it then moves into the follicle and interacts with B cells to produce a secondary lymphoid follicle.

Revision tip

Remember that T cells are migratory, they travel between the blood and the lymph node where they sample the range of MHC-peptide complexes present. If there is a good 'fit', that T lymphocyte receptor (TCR) is specific and the lymphocyte undergoes activation, clonal expansion and differentiation in the lymph node. It then exits via the efferent lymphatics and travels back to the site of inflammation in the affected tissue.

---

2. Spleen

The largest secondary lymphoid organ in the body, located in the upper abdomen.

- Capsulated.
- Not linked to the lymphatic system.
- Collects antigen from blood and responsible for immunity to blood-borne pathogens.
- Consists of red pulp (site of red blood cell destruction, rich in macrophages) and a lymphoid-rich white pulp (containing one quarter of the body's lymphoid cells).
- Lymphocytes enter via blood vessels and are evident as periarteriolar lymphoid sheaths (PALS).
- Lymphoid follicles containing B cells occur at intervals along the PALS.
- A marginal zone which contains unique populations of resident, non-circulating B cells and macrophages, is found at the interface of the PALS/follicles and red pulp.

3. Mucosa-associated lymphoid organs

- Organized lymphoid structures found in mucosal organs e.g. tonsils, adenoids, appendix, peyers patches (gut-associated lymphoid tissue, GALT).
- Nasal-associated lymphoid tissue.
- Bronchus-associated lymphoid tissue.

Key features of mucosal associated lymphoid organs

- Upper layer of specialized thin epithelial cells (M cells) which facilitate pathogen entry from the lumen of the mucosa.
- Distinct mucosal recirculation.

continued

- Contain organized T and B cell areas, macrophages and dendritic cells.
- Ideal microenvironment for the activation of T and B cells and the generation of adaptive immune responses.
- Not always static structures but may appear during infection/disappear on resolution.

Cells

- All white blood cells (WBC) are made in the bone marrow and then travel into the blood stream (Figure 1.8).
- The majority of WBC contribute to innate defences with the exception of lymphocytes, which are the only cell type responsible for adaptive immune responses.

1. White blood cells (polymorphonuclear cells, mononuclear cells—numbers and characterization) found in peripheral blood (typical adult values)

See also the table of **Normal adult blood cell counts** in the Glossary.

Polymorphonuclear cells (PMN)

- The neutrophil is the commonest white blood cell (approximately 60%; $2–8 \times 10^9$ cells/l).
  - Characterized by lobed nuclei and one of the polymorphonuclear cells (PMN) or granulocytes
  - Large numbers produced by the bone marrow every day with a very short half life (>7h)
  - Rapidly recruited to sites of inflammation (by the chemokine CXCL8 also known as IL-8)
  - Destroy pathogens by phagocytosis
  - Trap pathogens by releasing large neutrophil extracellular traps (NETs) composed of DNA fibres (netosis)
- Eosinophils are relatively rare PMN (approximately 2–3%; $\sim 0.5 \times 10^9$ cells/l).
  - Blood borne
  - Play a key role in defence against parasites
  - Release highly basic and cationic proteins (e.g. major basic protein, eosinophil cationic protein) from intracellular granules which are toxic to pathogens
  - Release cytokines which stimulate inflammation
  - Release pro-inflammatory mediators (e.g. leukotrienes, platelet activating factor; see Table 3.4)
  - Not very phagocytic
  - Implicated in the pathogenesis of allergy and asthma
- Basophils are rare PMN (approximately 0.5%; $<0.2 \times 10^9$ cells/l).
  - Blood borne
  - Play a key role in defence against parasites

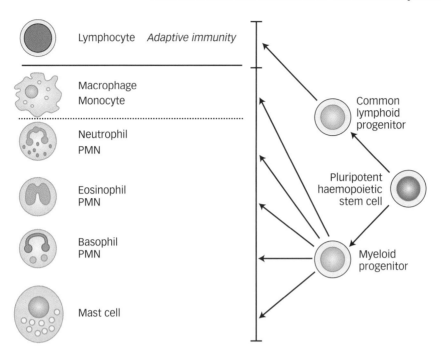

Figure 1.8 Cells of the immune system.

- ○ Express high affinity receptors for IgE
- ○ Rapidly release pre-formed inflammatory mediators (e.g. histamines, leukotrienes, cytokines; see Table 3.3 for more detail)
- ○ Implicated in the pathogenesis of allergy and asthma

Peripheral Blood Mononuclear cells (PBMC):
- Monocytes (approximately 4%; ~0.8 × 10⁹ cells/l).
  - ○ Blood borne
  - ○ Enter tissue and differentiate into macrophages
- Lymphocytes (approximately 24%; 1.6–4.8 × 10⁹ cells/l)
  - ○ B cells (10–15% of circulating lymphocytes)
    - ▪ Generally reside in B cell areas of lymph nodes (follicles)
    - ▪ Function to synthesize antibodies
    - ▪ Functionally heterogeneous populations
  - ○ T cells
    - ▪ CD4 helper T cells (50–60% of circulating lymphocytes)
      - ▫ Bind to class II MHC on specialized antigen-presenting cells
      - ▫ Secrete cytokines which help to activate other immune cells
      - ▫ Essential in the generation of adaptive immune responses

- □ Functionally heterogeneous populations exist (based on different cytokines they secrete (Chapter 2)
- □ Approximately 10% of CD4 helper cells down regulate immune responses and are referred to as Tregs
  - CD8 T cells (20–25% of circulating lymphocytes)
    - □ Bind to class I MHC expressed on all body cells
    - □ Can be activated to become cytotoxic T lymphocytes (CTL) which destroy infected/transformed body cells
    - □ Secrete cytokines (particularly γ-interferon)
    - □ Important in anti-viral and anti-tumour immune responses
- ○ Natural Killer Cells (10–15% of circulating lymphocytes)
  - Blood borne
  - Can be activated to kill infected/transformed body cells
  - Secrete cytokines (particularly γ-interferon)
  - Important in anti-viral and anti-tumour immune responses

Looking for extra marks?

Peripheral blood mononuclear cells (PBMC) can be isolated by density gradient centrifugation. Whole blood is layered onto a density gradient solution (e.g. 'lymphoprep' which has a density of 1.077 g/ml) and centrifuged. Red cells are more dense so are pelleted, the mononuclear cells (T and B cells, monocytes and NK cells) are lighter so float at the interface. They are sometimes referred to as the 'buffy coat'. Many immunological investigations are made with isolated PBMC, but they only reflect what is happening in the blood and not in tissue or lymph nodes.

2. Tissue resident white blood cells

- Macrophages
  - ○ Relatively long lived cells (e.g. months)
  - ○ Named according to their location (e.g. alveolar macrophages in the lungs, kupffer cells in the liver, mesangial cells in the kidneys, microglial cells in the brain)
  - ○ Kill pathogens by phagocytosis
  - ○ Release pro-inflammatory cytokines (e.g. TNFα, IL-1, IL-6)
  - ○ Remove dead (apoptotic) cells and contribute to the repair process
- Mast cells
  - ○ Express high affinity receptors for IgE
  - ○ Unique secretory system (degranulation)
  - ○ Rapidly release pre-formed inflammatory mediators (e.g. histamines, leukotrienes, cytokines; see Table 3.3 for more detail)
  - ○ Implicated in the pathogenesis of allergy and asthma

- Dendritic cells
  - Found at all barriers in close proximity to epithelial cells (including extending processes into the lumen of the mucosa)
  - Langerhans cells in the skin
  - Exist in an immature state in tissue—characterized by a high ability to internalize antigens
  - Drain to lymph nodes under steady state conditions which is increased in the presence of danger signals and inflammation
  - Differentiate to a mature state in lymph nodes, no longer capable of internalizing antigen but very effective at presenting antigen to T cells (express high levels of class II MHC and costimulatory molecules)
  - The only antigen-presenting cell (APC) that can activate a primary immune response
  - Functionally heterogeneous populations exist

Looking for extra marks?

Recent research has demonstrated that in addition to Natural Killer Cells there are also Natural Helper Cells. These are also referred to as 'Innate Lymphoid Cells' (ILC) and they are non-T non-B cells but secrete cytokines similar to helper T cell populations (and have been characterized as ILC1, ILC2 and ILC3). In addition, 'innate-like' lymphocytes (ILL) also exist. These are T or B cells which do express lymphocyte markers but their BCR/TCR variability may be more restricted, e.g. γδT cells, NKT cells, MAIT (mucosal-associated invariant T) cells and B1 cells.

Mediators

- Communication is essential in making effective immune responses.
- Soluble mediators carry messages around the body and modify the behaviour of other body cells.
- They also interact with each other to produce inflammatory cascades.
- Mediators can be classified according to their structure, function or source.
- Mediators produced by monocytes have been referred to as monokines, those produced by lymphocytes as lymphokines. However, these terms have been largely replaced by the general term cytokine (see Table 1.5 for the current list of interleukins).
- Cytokines can be defined functionally:
  - Immune effects, e.g. Interleukins (IL-1 to IL-37)
  - Chemotactic, e.g. chemokines (CXLC8 or IL8)
  - Pro-inflammatory, e.g. TNF-α, IFN-γ, IL-1β, IL-6
  - Anti-inflammatory, e.g. IL-10, TGFβ
  - Anti-viral effects, e.g. type I interferons (IFNα and IFNβ)
  - Haematological effects, e.g. colony stimulating factors (GM-CSF)
  - Cell biological effects, e.g. growth factors (TGFβ)

Structure, cells and mediators of the immune system

Name	Properties
IL1A interleukin 1, alpha	Pro-inflammatory cytokine (local and systemic). Induces the acute phase response. An important mediator in sterile inflammation (as an 'alarmin' or danger signal which is produced following necrotic cell death)
IL1B interleukin 1, beta	Pro-inflammatory cytokine (local and systemic). Induces the acute phase response. Synthesized as pro-IL1beta and not biologically active until processed by caspase-1
IL1F10 interleukin 1 family, member 10 (theta)	Member of the IL-1 family (also referred to as IL38)
IL1RN interleukin 1 receptor antagonist	Soluble molecule which binds to the IL-1 receptor but inhibits signalling. Anti-inflammatory
IL2 interleukin 2	T cell growth factor essential for T cell activation. Member of the common gamma chain family (cytokine receptor)
IL3 interleukin 3	Haematopoietic growth factor. Uses the same common beta subunit (cytokine receptor) as IL5 and GM-CSF
IL4 interleukin 4	T cell growth and differentiation factor (Th2). Member of the common gamma chain family (cytokine receptor)
IL5 interleukin 5	Th2 cytokine. Important in immune responses to helminths, IgE production and an increase in eosinophils. Uses the same common beta subunit (cytokine receptor) as IL3 and GM-CSF
IL6 interleukin 6	Pro-inflammatory cytokine (local and systemic). Induces the acute phase response
IL7 interleukin 7	T cell growth factor. Member of the common gamma chain family (cytokine receptor)
CXCL8 chemokine (C-X-C motif) ligand 8 (formerly IL8)	Chemotactic for neutrophils. First member of the chemokine family to be discovered. Often referred to as interleukin 8 (IL 8)
IL9 interleukin 9	T cell growth factor. Member of the common gamma chain family (cytokine receptor). Th2 cytokine. Important in immune responses to helminths, IgE production and an increase in eosinophils
IL10 interleukin 10	Anti-inflammatory cytokine
IL11 interleukin 11	Can stimulate haematopoiesis
IL12 interleukin 12	Differentiation factor for Th1 cells and activates NK cells. Made up of an alpha and beta chain (which are found in other IL-12 family members)
IL13 interleukin 13	Th2 cytokine. Important in immune responses to helminths, IgE production and an increase in eosinophils
IL14 interleukin 14	B cell growth factor
IL15 interleukin 15	T cell growth factor. Member of the common gamma chain family (cytokine receptor)
IL16 interleukin 16	Chemoattractant for T cells, promotes Th1 responses and inhibits Th2
IL17 interleukin 17	Pro-inflammatory, produced by Th17 effectors involved in destruction of extracellular pathogens and recruitment of neutrophils. Homodimer of IL17A or heterodimer with IL17F. Homologous family including IL17A, IL17B, IL17C, IL17D and IL17F
IL18 interleukin 18	Pro-inflammatory cytokine, member of the IL-1 family
IL19 interleukin 19	Member of the IL-10 family
IL20 interleukin 20	Member of the IL-10 family
IL21 interleukin 21	T cell growth factor. Member of the common gamma chain family (cytokine receptor). Differentiation factor for Th17 effectors.
IL22 interleukin 22	Member of the IL-10 family

IL23A interleukin 23, alpha subunit p19	Member of the IL-12 family (uses IL12beta chain). Differentiation factor for Th17 effectors
IL24 interleukin 24	Member of the IL-10 family
IL25 interleukin 25	Th2 cytokine. Important in immune responses to helminths, IgE production and an increase in eosinophils
IL26 interleukin 26	Member of the IL-10 family
IL27 interleukin 27 and IL30 (p38 subunit)	Member of the IL-12 family but thought to be anti-inflammatory
IL-28A, IL-28B, and IL-29	Member of the IL-10 family. Has homology with type I interferons and promotes anti-viral immune responses
IL31 interleukin 31	Th2 cytokine. Important in immune responses to helminths, IgE production and an increase in eosinophils
IL32 interleukin 32	Can upregulate pro-inflammatory cytokines
IL33 interleukin 33	Pro-inflammatory cytokine, member of the IL-1 family. Involved in Th2 responses to helminths (e.g. as an 'alarmin' released by damaged cells which activates mast cells)
IL34 interleukin 34	Stimulates monocyte proliferation and macrophage differentiation
IL35 interleukin 35	Member of the IL-12 family (uses IL12alpha chain)
IL36 interleukin 36	Member of the IL-1 family (IL36A, IL36B, IL36G)
IL37 interleukin 37	Pro-inflammatory cytokine, member of the IL-1 family

Table 1.5 Current list of interleukins

Source: HUGO Gene Nomenclature Committee at the European Bioinformatics Institute http://www.genenames.org/cgi-bin/genefamilies/set/601

Key features of cytokines

- All cytokines work through receptors which generate second messengers and lead to new gene transcription.
- Many cytokines are pleiotropic—one cytokine has multiple effects on one cell or multiple cell types.
- Several cytokines may exert similar functions ('redundant').
- Co-operative—they often act in a network, some cytokines enhance the production of others (synergy).
- Local and systemic—cytokines are small molecules and tend to act locally (**autocrine**, **paracrine**), however they can also act at distant sites (**endocrine**).

1. Cytokine receptors

- Cytokines mediate their effects via cytokine receptors.
- Cytokines bind to cytokine receptors and second messengers are generated.
- This leads to the activation of particular transcription factors and results in new gene expression.
- The common gamma chain (γC) is an example of a cytokine receptor that is shared amongst a number of related cytokine receptors (Figure 1.9). All these cytokines are involved in T cell proliferation and differentiation.

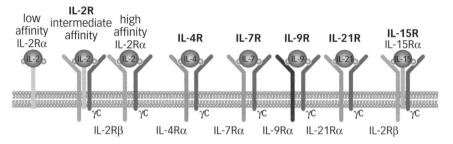

Figure 1.9 Common gamma chain cytokine receptor family.
Reprinted from *Journal of Allergy and Clinical Immunology,* **127**, Akdis et al., 'Interleukins, from 1–37, and interferon-γ: Receptors, functions, and roles in diseases', pp. 701–21, Copyright 2011, with permission from Elsevier.

Looking for extra marks?

Patients with single gene defects that lead to a failure to develop functional lymphocytes (i.e severe combined immunodeficiency SCID) are the first group of people who have been successfully treated with gene therapy. In particular, patients who lack this common gamma chain fail to produce any T cells or NK cells resulting in frequent and recurrent infections. This shows how important these cytokines are to the normal growth and differentiation of T cells. The disease is referred to as X-linked SCID as the common gamma chain is found on the X chromosome and the phenotype is recessive, so mainly expressed in boys. Clinical trials have shown that the correct copy of the gene can be transferred back into the patients' stem cells (using retroviral vectors) and reconstitute a functional immune system.

2. Chemokines

The immune system is dynamic and motile. **Chemokines** are responsible for the directional movement of leukocytes into tissues, and lymphoid organs.

Key features of chemokines

• Chemotactic cytokines which fall into four distinct families based on their structure:

  chemokine (C-C motif) ligand 1-28 (CCL1-28)

  chemokine (C-X-C motif) ligand 1-17 (CXCL1-17)

  chemokine (C-X3-C motif) ligand 1 (CX3CL1)

  chemokine (C motif) ligand 1 (XCL1)

- Chemokines exert their action by binding to transmembrane chemokine receptors (all 7 transmembrane G protein linked):

  chemokine (C-C motif) receptor 1-10 (CCR1-10)

  chemokine (C-X-C motif) receptor 1-6 (CXCR1-6)

  chemokine (C-X3-C motif) receptor 1 (CX3CR1)

  chemokine (C motif) receptor 1 (XCR1)

- Multiple chemokines can bind to a single receptor, e.g. CXCL9, CXCL10 and CXCL11 can all bind to CXCR3. CCL3, CCL4 and CCL5 all bind to CCR5. CCL5 can also bind to other receptors (CCR1 and CCR3).
- Constitutive chemokine secretion is responsible for maintaining physiological traffic of leukocytes to discrete tissue micro-environments.
- Inducible chemokine secretion contributes to the evolution of inflammatory responses *in vivo*.
- Chemokines bind to glycosaminoglycans in extracellular matrix (e.g. heparan sulfate) in tissue.
- Pro-inflammatory cytokines can increase chemokine production from a wide range of tissue cells (e.g. epithelial cells, endothelial cells, etc.) which will create a concentration gradient and lead to the directional movement of leukocytes towards the site of inflammation.

Looking for extra marks?

Many viruses use chemokine receptors to adhere to, and gain entrance to, body cells. Human immunodeficiency virus (HIV) binds to CD4 on target cells and uses chemokine receptors as a co-receptor. Different strains of HIV can be characterized on whether they are T cell tropic (bind to CXCR4) or macrophage trophic (bind to CCR5) on target cells. Interestingly, a null mutation in CCR5 (Δ32) which leads to a lack of expression on this receptor on body cells also confers resistance to HIV infection.

1.6 NOMENCLATURE

You may have noticed that immunologists don't speak in English, but in a series of letters and numbers. This is a challenge to students who have to learn this new 'language'. If you can understand the terminology you will be able to access the many fascinating concepts in immunology.

Key features of CD numbers

- CD refers to 'cluster of differentiation' and identifies cell surface molecules on immune (and other) cells which are identified by a group of **monoclonal antibodies**.

continued

Nomenclature

- A molecule may have been assigned a CD number before immunologists knew its function. It is simply because one or more antibodies have been identified that can bind to it.
- CD numbers are assigned by international agreement at workshops on 'Human Leukocyte Differentiation Antigens' (HLDA).
- Currently the list includes CD1 (a–e) to CD364. This may increase following future HLDA workshops.
- They are generally cell surface antigens (although some intracellular antigens have been given a CD designation).
- They are used as markers to identify or **phenotype** cells.
- There are many resources to help you identify the nature of a particular CD number (see also Table 1.6).

  http://www.sciencegateway.org/resources/prow/index.html

  (Protein Reviews On the Web PROW—very good but not updated.)

  http://www.hcdm.org/MoleculeInformation/tabid/54/Default.aspx

  (Human Cell Differentiation Molecules is an organization which runs HLDA Workshops and names and characterizes CD molecules.)

CD number	Biochemical features	Cellular expression	Function
CD3	Made up of δ (20kDa), ε (20kDa), γ chains (25–28kDa) and ζ chains (16kDa)	T cells, thymocytes ⇒used to identify T cells	Associated with the T cell antigen receptor (TCR) and contributes to T cell signalling and cellular activation
CD4	55kDa Transmembrane protein, member of the Immunoglobulin (Ig) superfamily domain containing	T helper cells, some thymocytes Some peripheral blood monocytes and tissue macrophages	Accessory molecule which aids helper T cells bind to class II MHC/peptide complexes and contributes to T cell signalling and activation Receptor for HIV gp120
CD8	Either a homodimer of two CD8α chains or a heterodimer of a CD8α and CD8β chain (32–34kDa)	Cytotoxic T cells and their precursors, some thymocytes	Accessory molecule which aids cytotoxic T cells bind to class I MHC/peptide complexes
CD14	53–55kDa Membrane bound glycosylated protein	All peripheral blood monocytes, most tissue macrophages and some granulocytes ⇒used to identify monocytes	Receptor for lipopolysaccharide (LPS) on gram negative bacteria
CD19	95kDa Transmembrane protein, member of the Ig superfamily domain containing	B cells ⇒used to identify B cells	Part of a co-receptor (with CD21 and CD81) which forms a complex with the B Cell antigen Receptor (BCR) and contributes to the signalling process
CD25	45kDa Transmembrane protein, can exist as a homodimer, heterodimer (with IL-2R β CD122) or tripartite receptor (with IL-2Rβ and common γ chain CD132)	T cells, B cells, monocytes ⇒used to identify activated cells ⇒expressed by a subset of CD4+ regulatory T cells (Tregs)	IL-2 receptor alpha Dimeric CD25 forms the low affinity IL-2 receptor (binds IL-2 but doesn't signal) The high affinity IL-2 receptor consists of IL-2α, IL-2β and common γ chain (binds IL-2 and signals T cell proliferation)

CD28	44kDa Transmembrane protein expressed as a homodimer, member of the Ig superfamily domain containing	T cells	Costimulatory molecule which binds to CD80 and CD86 on antigen-presenting cells. Provides signal 2 for T cell activation
CD34	105-120kDa Heavily glycosylated type I membrane protein (sialomucin)	Haematopoietic stem and progenitor cells. Some endothelial cells ⇒used to identify haematopoietic stem cells	Cell adhesion and signalling. Binds to CD62L (l-selectin)
CD40	48kDa Type I transmembrane protein	B cells, macrophages, dendritic cells. Some epithelial cells	Costimulatory molecule binds to CD40L (CD154) on activated helper T cells. Leads to B cell activation and differentiation
CD45	Long single chain type I transmembrane molecule. Multiple isoforms exist which are differentially spliced (CD45RA 205–220kDa, CD45RO 180kDa, CD45RB 190–220kDa)	All haematopoietic cells ⇒used to identify leukocytes/bone marrow derived cells ⇒CD45RA identifies naïve T cells ⇒CD45RO identifies activated or memory T cells	Intracellular tyrosine phosphatase which plays a key role in B and T cell signalling and activation
CD56	Transmembrane protein (135–220kDa). Multiple isoforms exist, member of the Ig superfamily domain containing	Natural Killer (NK) cells ⇒used to identify NK cells (CD3– CD56+ cells)	Adhesion molecule (neural cell adhesion molecule 1)
CD80 (also referred to as B7.1)	60kDa Transmembrane protein, member of the Ig superfamily domain containing	Activated B cells. Some activated T cells and macrophages	Costimulatory molecule expressed by antigen-presenting cells (APC) which provides signal 2 to T cells. Binds to CD28 (which leads to T cell activation) and CTLA4 (which can lead to activation-induced cell death at the end of the immune response)
CD86 (also referred to as B7.2)	80kDa Transmembrane protein	Dendritic cells, monocytes, activated B cells	Costimulatory molecule expressed by antigen-presenting cells (APC) which provides signal 2 to T cells. Binds to CD28 (which leads to T cell activation) and CTLA4 (which can lead to activation induced cell death at the end of the immune response)
CD127	52kDa (isoform 1) Transmembrane protein. Member of the Ig superfamily domain containing (4 Isoforms exist 34kDa, 30kDa, 29kDa)	Lymphocyte precursors, T cells ⇒not expressed in a subset of regulatory T cells (Tregs) which can be identified as CD4+ CD25+ CD127–	IL-7 receptor alpha Forms a heterodimer with the common gamma chain (CD132)

Table 1.6 Some key CD numbers to know

Revision tip

Make your own list to help you decode the language you need to use on your particular course.

 Check your understanding

Discuss the role of inflammation in the biology of disease (you may choose your own example of a 'disease'). (*Hint: This question is asking you to explain acute (local and systemic) inflammation. In a disease, there is likely to also be some element of chronic inflammation. You may find it useful to explain the pathology from a micro (histology) and macro (bigger picture) perspective. You should include the vascular changes, cellular events and activation (in local inflammation), the changes in plasma proteins and distant organs (in systemic inflammation) and the tissue remodelling (in chronic inflammation).*)

Explain the principles behind vaccination. Illustrate your answer with specific examples. (*Hint: This question is asking you to explain adaptive immune responses and particularly how the vaccine stimulates a primary immune response so that a rapid secondary response is made to a pathogen. Should include evidence of decrease in infectious diseases following implementation. More marks will be given for the use of relevant examples.*)

Summarize the key structures of the immune system and explain their functions. (*Hint: You should discuss the primary lymphoid organs (responsible for the production of all white blood cells and the maturation of lymphocytes) and secondary lymphoid organs (i.e. lymph nodes, spleen and mucosal associated lymphoid tissue) which are specialized microenvironments to bring antigen together with specific lymphocytes and provide the optimal conditions for activation.*)

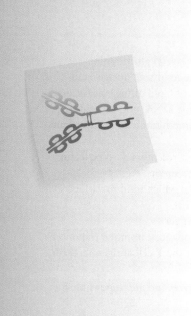

2 How is the Immune System Activated?

Immunologists think that the immune system has evolved to respond to harmful things that cause damage/cell death and are dangerous to the organism. This is called the 'danger hypothesis' and was first put forward over 20 years ago. You may also read about the 'self/non-self discrimination' model in text books. This states that the immune system responds to things that are different (or foreign), like pathogens or transplants.

Key concepts in recognition

- Recognition depends on receptors.
- Receptor binding results in signals being sent to the nucleus via the generation of second messengers which lead to new gene transcription and cellular activation.
- The key difference between the innate and adaptive immune responses is the way they recognize pathogens (using different types of receptors).
- The majority of white blood cells belong to the **innate** immune system and they possess many receptors which can recognize elements associated with pathogens.
  - These innate receptors tend to exploit differences between pathogens and the host, for example they recognize differences in the organization of sugars (e.g.

continued

peptidoglycan in bacterial cell walls contains N-acetyl glucosamine which is made up of regularly repeating glucose residues), nucleic acids (un-methylated cytidine-phosphate-guanosine or CpG dinucleotides are prevalent in bacterial but not vertebrate genomic DNA) and proteins (e.g. bacterial proteins often start with an N-formylmethionine or fMet residue, an amino acid not used by mammalian cells)

○ Many classes of innate receptors exist (scavenger receptors, C-type lectins, toll-like receptors, nod-like receptors, rig-like receptors, etc.)

○ They are **pattern recognition receptors** (**PRRs**) which bind to various pathogen-associated molecular patterns (**PAMPs**)

○ They are 'biased' to elements associated with danger

• Only lymphocytes (T and B) are responsible for adaptive immune responses and they possess only one type of receptor (either the T cell antigen receptor **TCR** or B cell antigen receptor **BCR**).

○ TCR and BCR are only expressed by lymphocytes and are responsible for adaptive recognition of pathogens

○ TCR and BCR are randomly rearranged receptors, each lymphocyte expresses a unique antigen receptor (with a different amino acid sequence at the antigen binding domain)

○ This random rearrangement has consequences—TCR and BCR which bind too strongly to self-proteins must be deleted (this is called self tolerance)

○ TCR and BCR are members of the immunoglobulin supergene family (i.e. they are made up from domains containing an anti-parallel beta sheet held together by a disulfide bond)

○ They are NOT 'biased' to pathogens (unlike innate receptors)

○ Each individual expresses many different TCR and BCR which represent a unique 'repertoire' of lymphocytes with ability to bind to pathogens

○ When individuals make an immune response to a pathogen, many different TCR and BCR will be activated

○ Different individuals will NOT respond in the same way to the same pathogen as we all have different TCR and BCR (and other immune response genes)

2.1 RECOGNITION BY THE INNATE IMMUNE SYSTEM

The **innate** immune system functions to 'sense' danger and send signals. The 'sensors' are specialized receptors which recognize structural elements of pathogens or products associated with cell damage/inflammation. These signals lead to the up-regulation of genes associated with inflammation, repair and the generation of adaptive immune responses.

Key features of the innate immune responses

- An ancient defence system present in all multicellular organisms—the receptors found in simple organisms are recognisable in more evolved organisms (e.g. humans).
- Widely distributed (**leukocytes** and all non-lymphoid cells).
- Rapid—forms the early phase of the host response.
- Not acquired—present in all individuals at all times.
- Does not change—no difference in response following repeated exposure to the same pathogen.
- Does not discriminate between pathogens, but responds to common microbial structures (for example).

Pathogen-associated molecular patterns/Pattern Recognition Receptors (PAMP/PRR) paradigm

Pathogen-associated molecular patterns (**PAMPs**) are recognized by pattern recognition receptors (**PRR**). These play a key role in innate host defences.

Key features of pattern recognition receptors (PRR)

- Recognize conserved molecular structures expressed by viruses, bacteria, fungi, protozoa, helminths, referred to as pathogen-associated molecular patterns (**PAMPs**).
- Recognize endogenous molecules associated with cellular stress and certain types of inflammatory cell death (**necrosis**, **pyroptosis**) referred to as damage-associated molecular patterns (**DAMPs**).
- Can be membrane bound, intracellular or secreted.
- Widely distributed on **leukocytes** and all body cells.
- Highly diverse and multiple different families exist (e.g. scavenger receptors, pattern recognition receptors, restriction factors, etc.).
- Evolved over millennia to recognize molecules unique to infectious organisms, e.g. exploit differences in cell wall/DNA/RNA structure.
- Lead to the generation of intracellular second messengers and the activation of transcription factors culminating in the transcription of new genes.

You may be surprised by how broad the range of key features is—but your immune system has to respond to many different types of pathogens that can attack any part of your body. They can be intracellular pathogens (e.g. all viruses) or extracellular (like most fungi, protozoa and helminths). Bacteria can be either intracellular (e.g. *Mycobacteria, Chlamydia, Salmonella, Legionella*) or extracellular pathogens (e.g. *Staphlococci, Streptococci, Enterobacteria, Clostridium, Listeria*).

> **Revision tip**
>
> Note that innate receptors represent the biology of evaluation through evolution. They are 'biased' to the enemy, i.e. pathogenic organisms.

Some examples are listed below:

1. Macrophage Mannose Receptor (MR also known as CD206)

- C-type **lectin** (Ca^{2+} dependent).
- Contains 8 carbohydrate recognition domains (CRD).
- Expressed mainly by **macrophages** and **dendritic cells.**
- Individual carbohydrate recognition domains have a low affinity for monosaccharides.
- Multiple carbohydrate recognition domains align with repeating mannose on pathogen cell walls to create high affinity, multivalent interactions.
- Can bind to repeating mannose sugars on *Mycobacterium tuberculosis, Streptococcus pneumonia, Yersinia pestis, Candida albicans, Pneumocystis carinii, Cryptococcus neoformans*, human immunodeficiency virus (HIV), influenza virus, dengue virus, and *Leishmania* species.
- Binding leads to enhanced uptake and antigen processing of **pathogens** (to stimulate **adaptive** immune responses).
- **Phagocytosis** leads to pathogen death and elimination (with the notable exception of *Mycobacterium Spp* although other pathogens can survive within phagocytes, e.g. *Leishmania, Histoplasma*).
- Scavenges unwanted/potentially harmful high mannose-linked glycoproteins from the circulation (so the MR is also referred to as a 'scavenger receptor').

2. Collectins

A family of C-type lectins which all have a collagen stalk, a neck region (which sets the angle of the carbohydrate recognition domain) and multiple units of trimeric carbohydrate recognition domains.

- Mannan binding lectin (MBL):
  - Soluble **acute phase protein** secreted by hepatocytes in the liver in response to systemic inflammation
  - Six carbohydrate recognition domains bind repeating sugars on many pathogens including HIV, ebola virus, influenza virus, *C. albicans, C. neoformans, Streptococci, Neisseria* and *Listeria* species
  - Can activate the lectin pathway of complement
- Surfactant protein A:
  - Secreted by alveolar epithelial cells in the lung, but also found in other mucosal sites

- Six carbohydrate recognition domains bind preferentially to repeating patterns of N-acetylmannosamine, then fucose, maltose, glucose, mannose
- Shown to bind to the major surface glycoprotein of *P. Carinii*, the outer membrane protein of *H .influenza*
- Binds to SP-A receptors on macrophages and facilitates **opsonization**
- Phagocytosis leads to pathogen death and elimination

3. Pentraxins

A family of plasma proteins with a distinctive cyclic pentameric structure. Each subunit binds to ligands in a Ca^{2+} dependent manner. They form part of the acute phase response to systemic **inflammation**.

- **C reactive protein (CRP)**:
  - Binds to phosphocholine residues on pathogens (e.g. *Streptococcus pneumonia, H. influenza, Neisseriae* species)
  - Can bind to polycations (e.g. poly l-lysine)
  - Binds to ligands on damaged host cells
  - Promotes phagocytosis by opsonization
  - Promotes complement activation (via C1q binding)
- Serum Amyloid component (SAP):
  - Binds to phosphoethanolamine and sugars (e.g. lipopolysaccharide on gram negative bacteria)
  - Can bind to polyanions (e.g. heparin and glycosaminoglycans, amyloid)
  - Can bind to necrotic/apoptotic cells
  - Promotes phagocytosis by opsonization
- Pentraxin 3 (PTX3):
  - Binds to *A. fumigatus, P. aeruginosa, K. pneumoniae, N. meningitides,* influenza virus
  - Promotes phagocytosis by opsonization

Revision tip

Remember opsonization is a trick the immune system plays over and over again. The idea is to coat a pathogen with a host protein, then have receptors for that host protein on phagocytes (e.g. macrophages and neutrophils). This will increase the affinity of the pathogen and drive it into these effective 'killers'. Other opsonins include complement proteins and antibodies.

Toll-like receptors (TLR)/inflammasome (nod-like receptors NLR)/retinoic acid-inducible gene I-like receptors (RLR) sensing

Signals from PRR are integrated by a highly conserved family of transmembrane receptors called **Toll-like receptors (TLR)** (Figure 2.1)

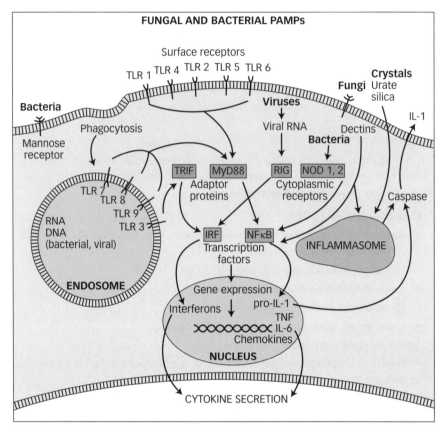

Figure 2.1 Pathogen-associated molecular patterns (PAMPs) are detected outside body cells by Toll-like receptors (TLRs) expressed on the plasma membrane. TLRs expressed on endosomal vesicles can detect viral PAMPs within the cytoplasm. Inflammasome complexes can detect intracellular PAMPs (e.g. from intracellular bacteria, fungi and viruses). Viral RNA can be also be detected by Rig-like receptors (RLR). Receptor binding leads to the activation of the NFκβ signal transduction pathway and the activation of pro-inflammatory cytokines and interferons (anti-viral responses). Damage-associated molecular patterns (DAMPs, e.g. urate) also bind to TLRs and inflammasome to activate innate immune responses.

Source: Infection and Immunity, Fourth Edition by John Playfair and Gregory Bancroft (2013). By permission of Oxford University Press. © John Playfair and Gregory Bancroft.

Key features of Toll-like receptors

- These molecules are highly conserved and found in all plants, invertebrates and vertebrates.
- They are expressed by immune cells including monocytes, macrophages and dendritic cells and also by tissue resident cells (e.g. mucosal epithelial cells, some endothelial cells).

- They are type 1 membrane proteins consisting of a recognition and signalling domain:
  - Extracellular ligand recognition domain (containing **l**eucine-**r**ich **r**epeats (LRR) and a cysteine-rich membrane-flanking region)
  - Intracellular signalling domain (**T**oll/**IL1 r**eceptor homology domain, TIR)
- Binding of pathogens to TLR leads to recruitment of 'adapter' molecules, the generation of second messengers and the activation of transcription factors, particularly NFκβ.
- NFκβ translocates to the nucleus and leads to the activation of immune response genes.
  - Promotes the production of pro-inflammatory cytokines
  - Promotes the activation of adaptive immune responses

There are 9 TLR in humans that can discriminate between different kinds of pathogens (Table 2.1). TLR10 is not thought to bind pathogens and may exert an anti-inflammatory function.

TLR are also reported to bind to endogenous ligands released by stressed or damaged tissue. These are referred to as damage-associated molecular patterns (**DAMP**s) or '**alarmins**' (Table 2.2). They may be released following certain types of cell death (**necrosis**, **pyroptosis**) or may be released from tissue following injury.

1. Inflammasomes

TLR are not the only molecules that sense danger and switch on immune response genes. An important family of intracellular complexes referred to as '**inflammasomes**' exist which can bind to PAMPs inside cells (Figure 2.1).

TLR	PAMP	Pathogen
TLR1	Diacylated and triacylated lipopeptides	Gram-positive bacteria Fungi
TLR2	Bacterial lipoproteins and other microbial cell wall components	
TLR6	Diacylated and triacylated lipopeptides	
TLR3	Double-stranded (ds) RNA	Viruses
TLR7	Single-stranded (ss) RNA	
TLR8	ssRNA	
TLR4	Lipopolysaccharide (LPS)	
TLR5	Bacterial flagellin	Gram negative bacteria
TLR9	Un-methylated cytidine-phosphate-guanosine (CpG) dinucleotides	Bacterial DNA

Table 2.1 List of Toll-like receptors and their ligands.

Recognition by the innate immune system

Endogenous agonist of TLR	Receptor
Components of extracellular matrix	
Heparan sulfate	TLR4
Hyaluronic acid	TLR4
Fibronectin extra-domain A	TLR4
Fibrinogen	TLR4
Biglycan	TLR2 and TLR4
Stress response molecules	
Heat-shock protein 60	TLR4
Heat-shock protein 70	TLR2 and TLR4
HMGB1 (high mobility group box 1)	TLR2 and TLR4
Immunomodulatory molecules	
β-Defensin	TLR1 and TLR2
Surfactant protein-A	TLR4
Chromatin–IgG complexes	TLR9
S100A8/A9	TLR4

Table 2.2 Some examples of DAMPs.

Key features of Inflammasomes

- A family of *intracellular* multi-molecular protein complexes that assemble in response to PAMPS/cell stress.
- Present in the cytosol and consist of a recognition and signalling domain:
  - ligand recognition domain (two main classes: containing either **n**ucleotide-binding **o**ligomerization **d**omains, NOD, and leucine-rich-repeat domains, or **py**rin and **HIN** domains, PYHIN)
  - Signalling: Pro-caspase 1 domain leads to the activation of the cysteine protease caspase-1
  - Leads to the processing and secretion of the proinflammatory cytokines interleukin-1β (IL-1β) and IL-18
- Promotes the production of pro-inflammatory cytokines.
- Promotes the activation of adaptive immune responses.
- Can cause inflammatory cell death (**pyroptosis**).

Looking for extra marks?

Mutations in inflammasomes are responsible for the majority of hereditary fever syndromes. They are characterized by fevers and inflammatory responses in the absence of antibody or T cell responses. For more information see Chapter 4, section 4.1, Auto-inflammatory diseases.

2. Sensors for viral nucleic acid (RNA, DNA) also exist in the cytoplasm:

- Helicases can bind dsRNA including **R**IG-I-**L**ike **R**eceptors (RLR) and MDA-5 (Figure 2.1).
- A number of DNA Sensors have been discovered (e.g. DAI, DDX41):
  - They have recognition and signalling domains like TLR and inflammasome
  - They lead to the activation of type I interferons (α and β interferon)
  - They promote anti-viral immune responses

Interferon (IFN) response

Production of type I interferons (**IFN-α** and **IFN-β**) is essential for antiviral immune responses. It is one of the consequences of recognition of viral elements by innate receptors (see earlier).

1. How are they produced?

- Innate recognition of viral RNA (e.g. by TLR3, TLR7, TLR8, RIG-1, MDA-5, see earlier) activates the Interferon Regulatory Factor System (IRFs).
- IRF3 and IRF 7 lead to transcription of IFN alpha and beta genes.
- All nucleated cells can secrete IFNα and IFNβ when infected by a virus.

2. What is their effect?

- Binding of IFNα and IFNβ to their receptors on uninfected neighbouring cells.
- Cellular Signalling (via STAT1, STAT2 and IRF9) and new gene transcription.
- Activation of many IFN-regulated genes (IRGs)/IFN-stimulated genes (ISGs).
- Increase host resistance to viruses by the production of many '**restriction factors**', e.g.:
  - Tetherin—binds to viral particles and prevents them budding from plasma membrane
  - TRIM5α/TRIMCyp—targets viral particles for degradation within the cytoplasm (by proteasome)

Revision tip

if you can remember the receptors that bind to antigen (or pathogen) then you will understand immunology more easily. The key difference between innate and adaptive immune responses is how they *recognize* pathogens. There are many innate cells and receptors. They generally bind to patterns on pathogens which are not found in the host. They therefore exploit differences in cell wall structure, organization of nucleic acid, etc. and are 'biased to the enemy'. This is very different from lymphocyte antigen receptors which are rearranged and randomly generated (see section 2.2).

2.2 RECOGNITION BY THE ADAPTIVE IMMUNE SYSTEM

Only **lymphocytes** (**B cells** and **T cells**) can mediate **adaptive** (or acquired) immune responses.

Key features of adaptive immune responses

- Only found in organisms with a backbone and a jaw.
- Mediated by lymphocytes (T and B cells).
- Enable us to make *specific* immune responses against anything (*diverse*) which result in *memory* (primary immune response).
- Re-exposure leads to *escalating responses* (secondary immune responses).
- Only two families of receptors exist: B cell antigen receptor (**BCR**) and T cell antigen receptor (**TCR**).
- Rearranged receptors are randomly generated and highly diverse.
- Self-reactive TCR are deleted in the thymus.
- Adaptive immune responses are generally required to clear an infection.

Revision tip

Don't forget that vaccination is one of the most effective public health measures which have been introduced to prevent disease. The vaccine induces a primary immune response which is (ideally) specific to a particular pathogen. Therefore first exposure to that pathogen will activate specific memory lymphocytes (fast secondary immune response) and prevent infection. Innate responses are also generated by including adjuvants in vaccine preparations in order to promote inflammation (and simulate danger). Vaccination leads to immunity.

Rearranged lymphocyte receptors

The BCR (Figure 2.2) and TCR (Figure 2.3) are membrane bound members of the immunoglobulin (Ig) superfamily which function to recognize **antigen** and initiate adaptive immune responses.

Key features of lymphocyte receptors

B cell receptor (BCR)	T cell receptor (TCR)
Surface immunoglobulin (mIgM)	Majority consist of alpha and beta chains (TCRαβ). Some have gamma and delta chains (TCRγδ)
Complexed with Ig α and Ig β chains in the plasma membrane	Complexed with CD3 gamma, delta, epsilon and zeta (γδεξ) chains
Recognize the three-dimensional shape (or tertiary structure) of an antigen.	Only recognize the primary structure of antigens—presented in the context of another molecule (peptide receptor called **MHC** or **major histocompatibility complex**)

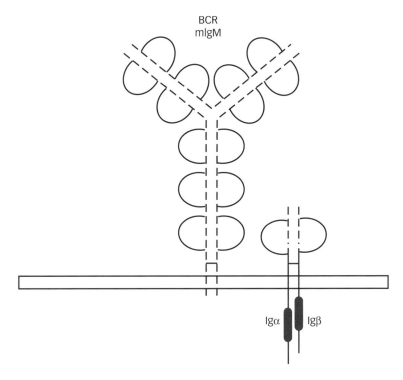

Figure 2.2 Illustration of the protein structure of the B cell antigen receptor (BCR) showing membrane bound IgM and associated Ig alpha and Ig beta chains (immunoreceptor tyrosine-based activation motifs ITAMs illustrated on the cytoplasmic domains).

Source: A. DeFranco and A. Weiss, 'Signal Transduction by T- and B- lymphocyte Antigen Receptors' in Ochs et al., *Primary Immunodeficiency Diseases: A Molecular and Genetic Approach*, 3rd edn (2013). By permission of Oxford University Press, USA.

1. What do the lymphocyte receptors bind to?

- BCR bind to the three dimensional (or tertiary) structure of an antigen (e.g. part of a pathogen):
  - ○ It can be protein, carbohydrate or lipid
- TCR do not bind directly pathogens:
  - ○ TCR bind to short fragments of peptide (primary structure) presented in a peptide receptor called MHC (major histocompatibility complex)
  - ○ **Class I MHC** are expressed on every body cell and present intracellular peptides to TCR
  - ○ **Class II MHC** are mainly expressed on specialized **antigen-presenting cells** and generally present extracellular peptides to TCR

TCR

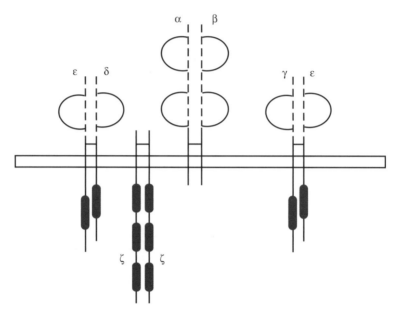

Figure 2.3 Illustration of the protein structure of the T cell antigen receptor (TCR) showing the alpha and beta chain complexed with CD3 gamma, delta, epsilon and zeta chains (immunoreceptor tyrosine-based activation motifs ITAMs illustrated on the cytoplasmic domains).

Source: A. DeFranco and A. Weiss, 'Signal Transduction by T- and B- lymphocyte Antigen Receptors' in Ochs et al., *Primary Immunodeficiency Diseases: A Molecular and Genetic Approach*, 3rd edn (2013). By permission of Oxford University Press, USA.

2. How are lymphocyte receptors rearranged?

Antigen receptors (BCR and TCR) are incredibly diverse. This diversity means our lymphocytes can respond to a very wide array of pathogens. This diversity is generated by a process called **somatic recombination.**

Key features of somatic recombination

- Multiple copies of gene segments (V Variable, J Joining, D diversity and C constant) which code for BCR and TCR proteins exist in the genome of immature lymphocytes. These immature lymphocytes do not express antigen receptors.
- Recombinase enzymes (**Recombination Activating Genes RAG-1 and RAG-2**) exist to recombine a single gene segment of each V(D)J and connect to a constant domain to make a functional receptor gene.

- When two gene segments have been selected at random by the RAG1/RAG2 complex and joined together, the intervening DNA is removed and lost from that lymphocyte.
- A highly regulated, sequential mechanism combines one Variable, one Diverse, and one Joining gene segment to generate a unique single gene V(D)J that will encode for a unique BCR or TCR variable region (the site which binds to pathogens).
- There are many combinations of V(D) and J which can lead to a high level of diversity.
- Recombination of lymphocyte receptor DNA occurs early in lymphocyte development and mature lymphocytes express rearranged receptors on their surface.
- This process produces enormous **lymphoid diversity** with lymphocytes possessing many highly variable rearranged antigen receptors (BCR, TCR).
- Lymphocyte receptor rearrangement is a random process which results in each individual generating very large and unique TCR and BCR 'repertoires'.
- B lymphocyte diversity takes place in the bone marrow.
- T lymphocyte diversity takes place in the thymus.

3. BCR rearrangement

- BCR genes are made up of heavy and light chains.
- Heavy chain genes are found on chromosome 14 and contain multiple V, D, J and C exons (Table 2.3).
- There are two kinds of light chain genes, κ kappa (chromosome 2) and λ lambda (chromosome 22). Light chain genes only contain V, J and C exons (Table 2.3).
- Rearranged BCR express either λ or κ light chains.
- They are commonly referred to as immunoglobulin (Ig) genes. **Antibody molecules** are essentially secreted BCR (for more information on the function of secreted antibodies, go to section 3.2 Destruction: adaptive effector mechanisms).

Segment	Light Chain		Heavy Chain
	Kappa (κ)	Lambda (λ)	Heavy (H)
Variable (V)	34–38	29–33	38–46
Diversity (D)	0	0	23
Joining (J)	5	4–5	6
Constant (C)	1	4–5	9

Table 2.3 Number of functional gene segments in human immunoglobulin genes. (Note: this will vary in different people due to genetic polymorphism.)

4. BCR Somatic hypermutation

During the course of an immune response, the BCR genes can undergo further mutation with the generation of even more receptor diversity. This leads to the generation of very high affinity antibodies specific to invading pathogens.

- Point mutations are introduced at a high frequency in dividing B cells (e.g. 10^3/cell division).
- This further diversifies the sequences of the V regions in BCR genes.
- Dividing B cells containing these point mutations are competing to BIND antigen in germinal centres (lymph nodes).
- Favourable mutations lead to changes which enable the daughter B cell to bind antigen with higher affinity than the original parent cell.
- Detrimental mutations fail to bind antigen and are no longer activated.
- **Affinity maturation**: the ability of B cells to make very high-affinity secreted antibodies which can bind more tightly to the antigen. This increase in BCR specificity during the course of an immune response will therefore improve the quality of the specific antibody effector functions (Table 2.4):
  - Sequence divergence produces a very wide range of functional Ig repertoires
  - This enables us to respond to the very wide range of pathogens we are exposed to throughout our lifetime and generate antibodies with increasing affinity as our immune response develops

Enzyme	Point mutation
Activation induced cytidine deaminase (AID)	Cytidine (C)→Uracil (U) by deamination
Uracil-DNA glycolase	U removed to create an abasic site on the DNA Random insertion of a nucleotide by DNA polymerase

Table 2.4 Mechanism of B cell hypermutation during the course of an immune response.

Affinity maturation takes place in specialized areas within lymph nodes called germinal centres (GC). They form about 6 days after primary immunization and are a focus of proliferating B cells and specialized helper T cells (T follicular helper cells, Tfh). These are highly dynamic structures and organized into areas where B cells are dividing (Dark Zone) and a Light Zone in which B cells are activated and selected based on their affinity for antigen. There is also a network of follicular dendritic cells within the light zone which retain/trap antigen long term and help to maintain the GC structure. **Affinity matured** GC B cells have been selected over time for their ability to bind to antigen. They contribute to long-lived humoral responses by differentiating into **plasma cells** and memory B cells.

5. TCR rearrangement

- TCR genes are made up of alpha and beta chains (most commonly) or gamma and delta chains (generally <5% of circulating T cells, also found in the gut mucosa).
- TCR alpha and delta genes are found on chromosome 14 and contain multiple V, D, J exons.
- TCR beta and gamma genes are found on chromosome 7 and contain multiple V and J exons (no D exons).
- Rearranged TCR express either $\alpha\beta$ or $\gamma\delta$ chains.
- Immature T lymphocytes which contain all the V(D)JC DNA sequences (Table 2.5) travel to the thymus in order to undergo rearrangement.
- They then undergo a selection process but no further mutation (unlike mature B cells).

6. Thymic selection of mature T cells

- The thymus is the site of T cell maturation.
- Immature T cells are called thymocytes and do not express rearranged TCR.
- Receptor rearrangement starts when thymocytes reach the subcapsular region of the thymus.

Segment	TCR alpha	TCR beta	TCR gamma	TCR delta
Variable (V)	70 +	52	14	8
Diversity (D)	0	2	0	3
Joining (J)	61	13	5	3
Constant (C)	1	2	2	1

Table 2.5 Number of gene segments in T cell receptors.

Source: Online Mendelian Inheritance in Man http://www.omim.org/

- Rearranged TCR are randomly generated so it is important to ensure they go through two checkpoints before joining the circulation:

  1. Is the rearranged TCR useful? Lymphocytes expressing TCR that can bind to self MHC with low affinity receive a survival signal. TCR that can't bind to self MHC die. This is *positive* selection.

  2. Is the rearranged TCR dangerous? Lymphocytes expressing TCR that bind to self MHC with high affinity receive a signal to die (apoptosis). This is *negative* selection.

- The majority of thymocytes die during the selection process (95%). It is referred to as **central tolerance.**

- The remaining 5% of lymphocyte express TCR with intermediate affinity for self MHC.

- This represents your T cell repertoire, and is highly diverse (estimated to contain 10^{16}–10^{18} unique TCR sequences).

Looking for extra marks?

Some people are born without a thymus (Di George's Syndrome), or have a genetic deficiency in the recombinase enzymes RAG-1/RAG-2. They cannot rearrange their TCR and have no mature T cells. This leads to severe combined immunodeficiency (SCID), see section 4.1.

2.3 ACTIVATION OF THE ADAPTIVE IMMUNE SYSTEM

Only lymphocytes (B and T cells) mediate adaptive immune responses. There are heterogeneous populations. The main cell types are summarized below.

- **Helper T cells** express the accessory molecule CD4 (which can bind to an invariant portion of MHC class II).

- **Cytotoxic T cells** express the accessory molecule CD8 (which can bind to alpha 3 domain of class I MHC).

- Regulatory T cells supress the activity of the other two populations and control immune responses.

- Conventional B cells with diverse BCR (sometimes referred to as B2 cells) which rely on T cell help for activation.

- **Plasma cells** are activated B cells which are producing antibodies (the Ig molecule released has exactly the same specificity as the membrane bound BCR).

- Unconventional B cells with less diverse BCR (referred to as B1 cells) which are less dependent on T cell help for their activation.

- If these lymphocytes have never been activated, they are referred to as **naive** (or virgin) **lymphocytes.**

Antigen presentation

- T cells are only activated in the presence of **antigen-presenting cells (APC).**
- These present a small part of the pathogen (peptide of 8–24 amino acids held in the peptide receptors MHC) to the TCR.

1. What is MHC?

- MHC are peptide receptors.
- There are two classes of MHC:
  - **Class I MHC** (comprised of an α chain non-covalently attached to $\beta2$ microglobulin, Figure 2.4)
  - **Class II MHC** (comprised of an α and β chain, Figure 2.4)
- Similar tertiary (three dimensional) structure, both types of MHC have a peptide binding groove (2 alpha helices above a beta pleated sheet, Figure 2.5).
- MHC proteins don't fold correctly/transit to the cell membrane unless a peptide is bound within its groove.
- MHC in humans are called human leukocyte antigens (HLA):
  - Class I MHC are HLA A, B and C
  - Class II MHC are HLA DR, DP and DQ
  - Co-dominant expression of maternal and paternal HLA so each body cell expresses 2 copies of HLA-A, 2 copies of HLA-B and 2 copies of HLA-C (i.e. 6 different class I MHC)

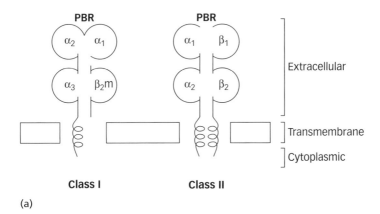

(a)

Figure 2.4 (a) Illustration of the protein structure of the Major Histocompatibility Complex (MHC) molecules showing the peptide-binding region (PBR). (b) Ribbon diagram of the crystal structure of class I MHC. (c) Ribbon diagram of the crystal structure of class II MHC. Figure 2.4a Reproduced with permission of Annual Review of Genetics, Volume 32 © 1998 by Annual Reviews, http://www.annualreviews.org; Ribbon diagrams courtesy of Dr Sheikh Naeem Shafqat, UBD.

Activation of the adaptive immune system

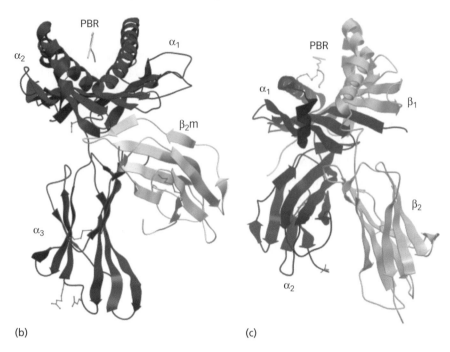

(b)   (c)

Figure 2.4 Continued

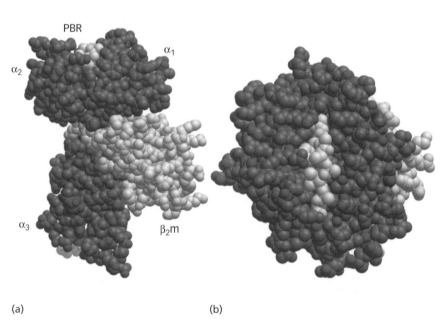

(a)   (b)

Figure 2.5 Space filling model of the crystal structure of MHC class I peptide complex (a) side view (b) top view.

Courtesy of Dr Sheikh Naeem Shafqat, UBD.

- o Specialized antigen-presenting cells (plus some endothelial cells and epithelial cells) express three maternal and three paternal class II alpha and beta alleles (i.e. up to 12 different class II MHC)
- o They are the most **polymorphic** genes within the human population and the chance of you having the same MHC genotype as anyone else is extremely small (see Figure 4.6)
- Different MHC will bind a different spectrum of peptides (depending on the specific peptide-binding properties of each allele).

2. How are peptides presented by class I MHC?

- Class I MHC display intracellular peptides (~ 9 amino acids long).
- All cytoplasmic proteins are degraded by proteasome (a complex of proteases that degrades proteins into short peptide fragments; see Figure 2.6).
- 9 amino acid peptides are actively transported into the endoplasmic reticulum by the Transporter associated with Antigen Processing (TAP) by an active process dependent on ATP.
- Suitable peptides are bound by the newly synthesized class I MHC which are then transported to the plasma membrane.
- Different class I MHC can bind to a different spectrum of peptides depending upon the presence of certain anchor residues, e.g.:
  - o HLA A2 binds to peptides with a leucine in position 2 and 9
  - o HLA B27 binds to peptides with an arginine in position 2
- Normally self peptides are presented in self MHC (in the absence of infection).
- If the cell is infected, then the pathogen is processed (by proteasome) and peptide fragments from it will be presented in class I MHC molecules.
- Different people express different class I MHC (HLA) so will present different fragments of a pathogen to their TCR.
- CD8 T cells bind to MHC class I/peptide complexes (Figure 2.7).

3. How are peptides presented by class II MHC?

- Class II MHC generally display extracellular peptides (~22–24 amino acids long).
- Newly synthesized class II MHC alpha and beta chains bind a third invariant chain in the endoplasmic reticulum. This prevents any other peptides from binding (Figure 2.6).
- This complex enters an endosome which will eventually merge with the endocytic pathway.
- Invariant chain is degraded by proteases inside this vesicle leaving a small portion remaining in the class II peptide groove (CLIP **Cl**ass II associated **i**nvariant chain **p**eptide).
- Pathogens are internalized and degraded by the endocytic pathway, and the vesicles containing class II MHC/CLIP complexes merge with vesicles containing pathogen-derived peptides.

Activation of the adaptive immune system

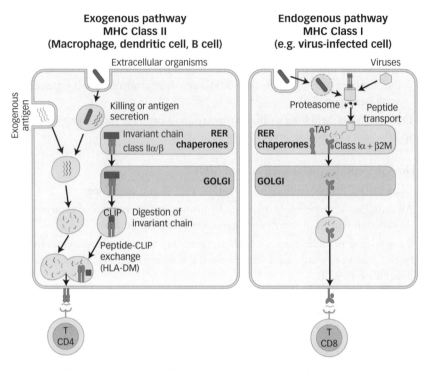

| Exogenous pathway
MHC Class II
(Macrophage, dendritic cell, B cell) | Endogenous pathway
MHC Class I
(e.g. virus-infected cell) |

Figure 2.6 Schematic illustration of the class I and class II peptide-loading pathways. Class II MHC is generally expressed on specialized antigen-presenting cells. Extracellular or exogenous peptides enter the cytoplasm via an endosomal pathway and merge with newly synthesized class II MHC stabilised by an invariant chain. The invariant chain is removed and replaced by extracellular peptide with the aid of HLA-DM. Once the class II MHC/peptide complex has been produced it is transported to the plasma membrane. CD4 helper T cells bind to class II MHC/peptide complexes. Class I MHC expresses intracellular or endogenous peptides. The proteasome enzyme complex within the cytoplasm degrades intracellular proteins into small peptides which are actively transported into the endoplasmic reticulum (ER) by ATP-dependent transporters (TAP). In the case of a viral infection, viral proteins will be also degraded by proteasome and transported in the ER. Newly synthesized class I MHC molecules bind to particular peptides and form a stable complex which is then transported to the plasma membrane. CD8 T lymphocytes bind to class I MHC/peptide complexes.

Source: Infection and Immunity, Fourth Edition by John Playfair and Gregory Bancroft (2013). By permission of Oxford University Press. © John Playfair and Gregory Bancroft.

- A molecule called HLA-DM catalyses the release of CLIP from the peptide binding groove and its replacement with a pathogen-derived peptide.
- The class II MHC peptide complex is then transported to the plasma membrane.
- Different class II MHC molecules will display a different spectrum of peptides based on the position of certain anchor residues which can bind pockets in the MHC class II peptide binding groove.
- CD4 T cells bind to MHC class II/peptide complexes (Figure 2.7).

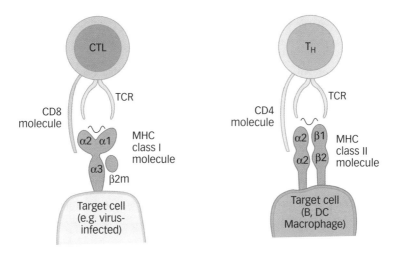

Figure 2.7 Cytotoxic T lymphocytes (CTL) use CD8 to bind to a monomorphic domain on class I MHC molecules. This helps to stabilise the interaction between CTL and target cells thereby enabling the TCR to bind to the specific MHC/peptide complex. Helper T cells (Th) use CD4 to bind to class II MHC to stabilise the interaction with antigen-presenting cells (APC) so that the TCR can bind to class II MHC/peptide complexes on the cell surface.

Source: Infection and Immunity, Fourth Edition by John Playfair and Gregory Bancroft (2013). By permission of Oxford University Press. © John Playfair and Gregory Bancroft.

Revision Tip

Why are there so many different types (or alleles) of MHC in the population? MHC polymorphism means there is great diversity in how we process pathogens and present pathogen peptides to our T cells. Therefore we make different immune responses to the same pathogen! Pathogens can mutate far faster than humans, and if they want to survive in a human host, they need to avoid recognition and destruction. However, mutations that may be beneficial to a pathogen in one situation may have no advantage in another.

Revision tip

Don't forget—MHC are peptide receptors. MHC class I (HLA A, B, C in humans) are expressed on all nucleated body cells, express peptides derived from inside the cell (e.g. either self peptides, or in the case of a viral infection, viral peptides). CD8 can also bind class I and is the co-receptor for cytotoxic T cells. MHC class II (HLA DR, DP and DQ in humans) are generally expressed by specialized antigen-presenting cells. They generally express peptides derived from outside the cell. CD4 binds to class II MHC and is the co-receptor for helper T cells.

Activation of the adaptive immune system

Costimulation

1. How are T cells activated?

Danger signals upregulate immune response genes that enable T and B lymphocytes to be activated. This is a tightly controlled process (Table 2.6 and Figure 2.8).

- Activation of helper T lymphocytes is the first step to induce adaptive immune responses.
- Three signals are required to activate a T helper (Th) cell.
- These are provided by an antigen-presenting cell (APC).
- The most potent APC that can activate a naive T cell is a dendritic cell.
- This generally takes place in secondary lymphoid organs (e.g. lymph nodes, spleen, Peyer's Patches).

2. T cell signalling

A highly regulated series of events leads to the creation of an activated T cell receptor complex and ultimately the activation of that specific T cell. This leads to the clonal expansion of that particular T cell (Figure 2.9).

- Signal 1 (specific binding of a TCR to an appropriate MHC/peptide complex) leads to the phosphorylation of the intracellular domains of CD3 ($\gamma\delta\varepsilon$ and ξ chains contain **immuno-receptor tyrosine-based activation motifs ITAMs**).
- Co-receptors contribute to the signal, e.g. CD45 will dephosphorylate the cytoplasmic domain of CD4 enabling it to contribute to the phosphorylation of ITAMs and generation of the intracellular signal.

Function	Molecules	Key point
Signal 1	TCR binding to a specific MHC/peptide complex on an APC	Responsible for the specificity of adaptive immune responses
Signal 2	**Costimulation**, e.g. CD28 (T cell) binding to CD80 or CD86 (also known as B7-1 and B7-2) on an APC	Only upregulated following activation of APC (e.g. by a DANGER signal)
Signal 3	**Cytokines**, e.g. IL-12/Interferon-γ induce T helper 1 responses IL4 induce T helper 2 responses	Determine the type of adaptive immune response that develops
Adhesion molecules	**Integrins** (e.g. LFA-1 or αLβ1) binding to **Ig superfamily** adhesion molecules (e.g. ICAM-1)	Tight adhesion of the T cell to the APC
Signalling molecules	CD3 (complexed with the TCR), CD4 (binds to MHC class II, has kinase activity when activated), CD45 (a phosphatase, activates CD4 signalling) are anchored on a lipid raft together with TCR/CD28 (signal 1/signal 2)	Contribute to the generation of second messengers and **nuclear factors** which lead to lymphocyte activation

Table 2.6 Summary of T cell activation.

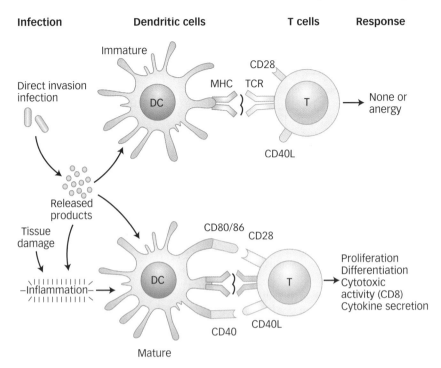

Figure 2.8 T cell activation is tightly controlled. If a TCR binds to a specific MHC/peptide complex presented by an antigen-presenting cell (e.g. a dendritic cell, DC) in the absence of inflammation, then the costimulatory molecules (CD80/86 or CD40) are not upregulated. This does not activate the T cell fully, and may result in a specific hypo-responsiveness or anergy. Inflammation stimulates production of pro-inflammatory cytokines and induces up-regulation of costimulatory molecules (e.g. CD80/CD86 and CD40). This provides both signals required for T cell activation (1) specific interaction of the TCR and MHC/peptide complex and (2) costimulation. This results in the T cell proliferation, differentiation and effector functions which ultimately should resolve the infection.

Source: Infection and Immunity, Fourth Edition by John Playfair and Gregory Bancroft (2013). By permission of Oxford University Press. © John Playfair and Gregory Bancroft.

- This enables a protein kinase, ZAP-70 to bind to the cytoplasmic domains of the T cell receptor complex and then recruit additional signalling molecules to this activated T cell receptor complex (e.g. linker of activated T cells LAT, SLP-76) and importantly a key signalling molecule phospholipase C-γ (PLC-γ).
- Signal 2 (costimulation) leads to the activation of PI 3 Kinase which activates PLC-γ and enables the generation of second messengers diacylglycerol (DAG) and inositol 1,4,5-triphosphate (IP_3).
- This leads to an increase in intracellular calcium which binds to calmodulin and activates a protein phosphatase calcineurin.
- An inactivated transcription factor (**nuclear factor of activated T cells NFAT**) is dephosphorylated and transits into the nucleus to bind to promotor sites.

Activation of the adaptive immune system

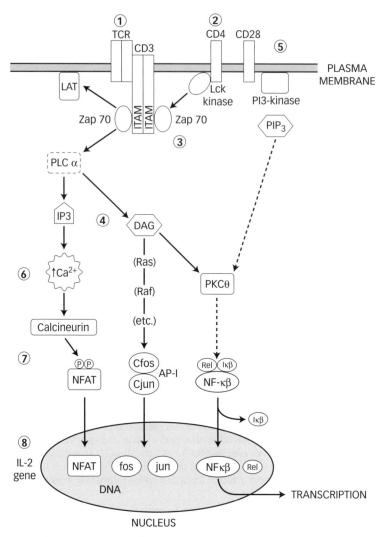

Figure 2.9 Schematic summary of the T cell activation pathway.

1. T cell antigen receptor (TCR) binds to specific MHC-peptide complex. Accessory molecules CD4 and CD8 also contribute to MHC binding and signalling.

2. In this example, CD4 also binds to class II MHC and helps stabilise TCR: MHC-peptide interaction. If binding is specific then CD3 zeta chains are phosphorylated at immuno-receptor tyrosine-based activation motifs (ITAMs) with the aid of lck kinase associated with CD4.

3. Tyrosine kinase Zap 70 can then bind these phosphorylated residues and go onto phosphorylate other proteins including scaffold protein 'linker of activated T cells (LAT)' and ultimately activate signalling molecule phospholipase C-γ (PLCγ).

4. This leads to generation of second messengers including <u>inositol 3 phosphate (IP3)</u> and <u>diacycglycerol (DAG),</u> which ultimately activate a number of transcription factors (AP-1 and NF-κβ; AP-1 is a dimer of fos and jun; NF-κβ is normally held in an inactive state by binding to an inhibitory protein, Iκβ).

5. Costimulatory signals from CD28 signalling are mediated through <u>phosphoinositide 3-kinase (PI-3 kinase),</u> which leads to generation of <u>phosphatidylinositol (3,4,5)-trisphosphate (PIP$_3$).</u>

6. This leads to an increase in <u>intracellular calcium (iCa^{2+})</u> which activates <u>calcineurin,</u> a protein phosphatase which then dephosphorylates inactive transcription factor <u>NFAT (nuclear factor of activated T cells)</u> enabling it to translocate to the nucleus.

7. Three key transcription factors are activated by the signal transduction pathway (NFAT, AP-1 and NF-κβ) which act in the nucleus to stimulate gene transcription leading to the differentiation, proliferation and effector functions of T cells.

8. <u>Interleukin 2</u> is a key T cell growth factor which is activated by these three transcription factors.

- DAG and IP3 also activate other transcription factors (e.g. NFκB and AP-1).
- New gene transcription, particularly IL-2 (a T cell growth factor) and its receptor lead to cell proliferation and differentiation.
- At the end of the immune responses, inhibitory costimulatory molecules are expressed (e.g. the intracellular molecule CTLA4 translocates to the cell membrane) which bind with higher affinity to CD80/CD86 on the APC. This blocks antigen presentation and switches off the immune response.
- Signal 1 in the absence of signal 2 leads to **anergy**, the specific T cell is switched off (hypo-reactive) and more difficult to activate.

Looking for extra marks?

People with defects in this signalling pathway (e.g. ZAP-70 deficiency) cannot activate their T cells and are unable to make adaptive immune responses. Consequently, they have a severe combined immunodeficiency.

Immunosuppressive drugs target this signalling pathway. For example cyclosporin A (CsA) and tacrolimus (also known as FK-506) block calcineurin and so prevent the activation of NFAT-dependent genes. They were developed to inhibit the rejection of solid organ transplants (e.g. kidney) but are also used to treat autoimmune diseases and inflammatory skin conditions.

Looking for extra marks?

There are two key 'check points' for immune activation. The first is CTLA4, an intracellular 'negative regulator' of immune activation. It has a higher affinity for the costimulatory molecules CD80/C86 expressed on antigen-presenting cells. It

continued

is presented on the surface of activated cells at the end of the immune response and functions to down regulate immune responses. Scientists have created a useful 'signal 2' blocker by attaching the CTLA4 molecule to an Ig domain (CTLA4-Ig) which can be used to block costimulatory signals and therefore inhibit immune responses. The second is PD-1, which is expressed on the surface of lymphocytes and appears to attenuate the activation signal and can cause the specific response to switch off (tolerance). CTLA4 and PD-1 can therefore inhibit immune responses. Monoclonal antibodies which block CTLA4 and PD-1 seem to reverse the immunosuppression observed in cancer tissue and are a promising immunotherapy.

3. How are B cells activated?

The process has some similarities to T cell activation (Figure 2.10 and Table 2.7):

- BCR Igα and Igβ chains contain ITAMs.
- Binding of specific antigen to BCR will cross-link the receptor, activating tyrosine kinases which phosphorylate these ITAMs in the cytoplasmic domains of the BCR.
- A B cell co-receptor (CD19, CD21, CD81) forms a complex with the BCR and contributes to the signalling process.
- Complement (C3)-coated pathogens will bind CD21 (also known as complement receptor 2) and be localized to the BCR complex.
- B cells do not express ZAP-70 but a similar tyrosine kinase called Syk which binds to phosphorylated Igβ and becomes activated.
- This leads to activation of a key signalling molecule phospholipase C-γ (PLC-γ) and the generation of second messengers DAG and IP_3.
- The transcription factors NFAT, NFκB and AP-1 are activated, translocate to the nucleus and bind to the promotor sites of particular genes leading to B cell proliferation and differentiation.
- T cell help is generally needed to fully activate B cells and enable them to differentiate into antibody-producing plasma cells.
- T-independent antibody production can occur when innate receptors on the B cell are also activated (e.g. TLR).

Looking for extra marks?

People with defects in this signalling pathway (e.g. B cell specific Tec kinase Bruton's tyrosine kinase Btk deficiency, located on the X chromosome) cannot activate their B cells. They cannot synthesize antibodies and have X-linked agammagloubinaemia. Consequently, they have a severe combined immunodeficiency (see section 4.1).

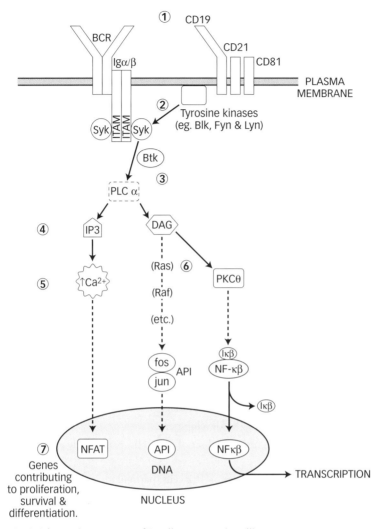

Figure 2.10 Schematic summary of B cell receptor signalling.

1. B cell antigen receptor (BCR) is cross-linked when bound by specific antigen. This brings together three protein tyrosine kinases (Blk, Fyn and Lyn) which are associated with B cell co-receptor complex (CD19, CR2 and CD81).

2. BCR associated Igα and Igβ chains contain immuno-receptor tyrosine-based activation motifs (ITAMs), which are phosphorylated by these tyrosine kinases.

3. The tyrosine kinase Syk then binds to these phosphorylated residues, activating a B cell specific kinase Bruton's tyrosine kinase (Btk), leading to activation of key signalling molecule phospholipase C-γ (PLCγ)

continued

Activation of the adaptive immune system

4. This leads to generation of second messengers including <u>inositol 3 phosphate (IP3)</u> and <u>diacycglycerol (DAG)</u>, which ultimately activate a number of transcription factors.

5. <u>IP3</u> leads to an increase in intracellular calcium <u>(iCa^{2+})</u>, which activates transcription factor <u>NFAT</u> (nuclear factor of activated T cells) in a calcineurin-dependent mechanism enabling it to translocate to the nucleus.

6. DAG activates <u>protein kinase C</u>, which leads to the activation of two other transcription factors: <u>AP-1</u> (a dimer of fos and jun) and <u>NF-κβ</u> (inhibited by Iκβ).

7. Ultimately three key transcription factors (NFAT, AP-1 and NF-κβ) are activated by the signal transduction pathways which result in new gene transcription leading to B cell differentiation, proliferation and survival.

4. How does the immune system generate the appropriate kind of immune response?

- Helper T cells produce cytokines which help other immune responses (Figure 2.11 and Table 2.8).
- Different helper T cells produce different cytokines according to the circumstances.
- Signal 3 from an APC will differentiate helper T cells with different effector functions.
- Differentiated helper T cells can be identified by the activation of a master transcription factor which contributes to their function.
- Not all Th cells secrete all the cytokines associated with any particular subset.
- Th1 and Th2 subsets are thought to be terminally differentiated.
- Th1 cytokine IFNγ inhibits Th2 development.
- Th2 cytokine IL-10 inhibits Th1 development.
- Th17 were shown to be a unique subset of Th1 cells, particularly associated with inflammatory diseases.
- Th9 appear to be a unique subset of Th2 cells, particularly associated with allergic diseases.
- Th17 and (induced) Tregs are not fixed in a particular phenotype and can change depending on the signals in the tissue (high TGFβ promotes Treg development, low TGFβ and IL-6, e.g. following systemic inflammation promotes Th17 differentiation).

Function	Molecules	Key point
Signal 1	BCR binds to specific antigen, then processes and presents it to a specific helper T cell (via its class MHC/peptide complex)	Responsible for the specificity of adaptive immune responses
Signal 2	Costimulation e.g. CD40 (B cell) binding to CD40L on a helper T cell	A specific helper T cell is required to activate a specific B cell
Cytokines	IL-4, IL-5	Stimulate differentiation into plasma cells and antibody production

Table 2.7 Summary of B cell activation.

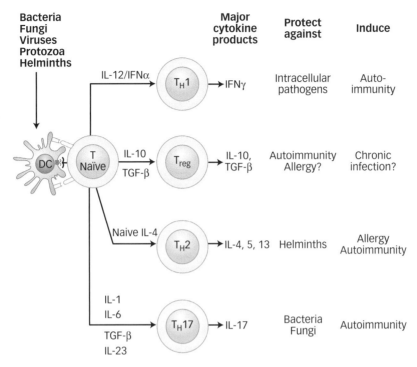

Figure 2.11 The activation of a naive helper T cell requires three signals from a professional antigen-presenting cell (dendritic cell DC): (1) specific interaction of the TCR with the class II MHC/Peptide complex, (2) costimulation, (3) cytokine signal. The type of infection will stimulate a different response in tissue. This influences the maturation of the DC which will travel to the lymph node to activate T cells. For example, intracellular pathogens (e.g. viruses) will induce IL12 upregulation in DC and induce a Th1 immune response. These helper cells will activate CTL which will travel back to the tissue and specifically destroy the infected cells. Helminths will induce IL4 secretion in DC and induce a Th2 immune response. This will activate IgE antibodies and mast cell/eosinophils in order to promote the expulsion of the helminth.

Source: Infection and Immunity, Fourth Edition by John Playfair and Gregory Bancroft (2013). By permission of Oxford University Press. © John Playfair and Gregory Bancroft.

Looking for extra marks?

Immune responses are polarized, and helper T cell responses are characterized by a spectrum of different cytokines. Leprosy is a good example of disease where the outcome is influenced by the type of helper T cell response (Figure 2.12). It is caused by the bacterium *Mycobacterium leprae,* which we find very difficult to destroy (it is resistant to killing by macrophages). There are two forms of leprosy: tuberculoid and lepromatous. Tuberculoid leprosy is characterized by Th1 cytokines (IL-2, IFNγ and LT) and the patient is controlling the bacteria by production of granulomas, and this is viewed as a 'healing' phenotype. In contrast, lepromatous leprosy is dominated by Th2 cytokines (IL-4, IL-5 and IL-10) and is associated with high infectivity, disseminated infection and multiple skin lesions.

Activation of the adaptive immune system

Signal 3	T helper cell	'Helper' cytokines produced	Master transcription factor	Function
IL-12; Interferon-γ	Th1	IL-2, IFNγ, lymphotoxin α (Lfα), TNFα	T-bet	Cell mediated immunity and inflammation. Associated with macrophage activation. Linked to autoimmunity and transplant rejection
IL-4	Th2	IL-4, IL-5, IL-9, IL-13, IL-10, IL-25	GATA-3	Antibody mediated immunity, associated with mast cell activation. Important in immune responses to helminth infections. Linked to allergy and asthma
TGFβ, IL-6, IL-21, IL-23	Th17	IL-17, IL-6	RORγT	Pro-inflammatory, associated with many disease states (e.g. transplant rejection, autoimmunity)
TGFβ	Treg (sometimes called Th3)	IL-10, TGFβ	FOXP3	Anti-inflammatory, reduce immunopathology associated with infection, associated with cancer

Table 2.8 Summary of cytokine signals that can polarize helper T cell responses.

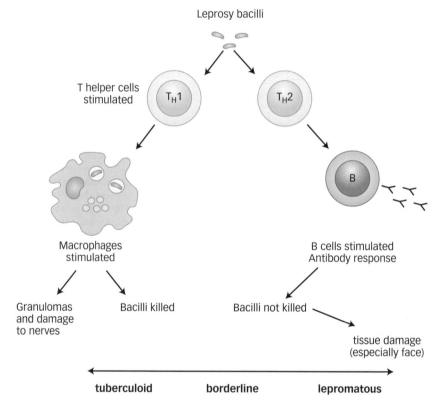

Figure 2.12 Illustration of how M. leprae can induce either a Th1 immune response which contains the infection and leads to granuloma formation (tuberculoid leprosy) or a Th2 immune response which stimulates antibody production. This response does not contain the bacteria leading to lepromatous leprosy which is characterized by disseminated infection and significant tissue damage.

Source: Infection and Immunity, Fourth Edition by John Playfair and Gregory Bancroft (2013). By permission of Oxford University Press. © John Playfair and Gregory Bancroft.

Clonal selection and differentiation

Once a lymphocyte binds to a pathogen, and receives a costimulatory signal, the next stage is to make multiple copies of this specific lymphocyte in order to generate an army of effectors that can bind specifically to the same pathogen and ultimately destroy it.

1. Clonal selection (McFarlane Burnett)

- Lymphocytes display surface receptors (TCR/BCR) for specific antigens.
- Lymphocyte populations have pre-existing randomly generated diverse antigen receptors (Figure 2.13).

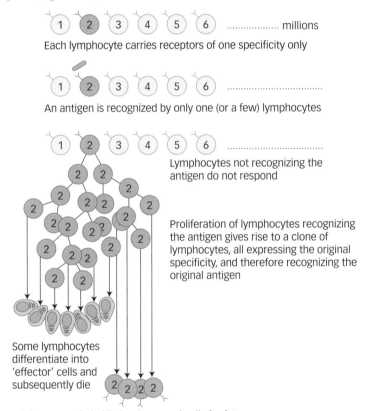

Each lymphocyte carries receptors of one specificity only

An antigen is recognized by only one (or a few) lymphocytes

Lymphocytes not recognizing the antigen do not respond

Proliferation of lymphocytes recognizing the antigen gives rise to a clone of lymphocytes, all expressing the original specificity, and therefore recognizing the original antigen

Some lymphocytes differentiate into 'effector' cells and subsequently die

Others remain behind as 'memory' cells for future use

Figure 2.13 Schematic illustration of lymphocyte receptor diversity and clonal selection of specific lymphocytes following receptor engagement. Every individual has a highly diverse repertoire of lymphocytes (B and T) with many different antigen receptors. A lymphocyte bearing a useful receptor that can bind to an antigen is stimulated to proliferate (in secondary lymphoid tissue) and produces many identical antigen-specific daughter cells (clones) which differentiate into effector cells. The majority will undergo activation-induced cell death at the end of the immune response. Some of the daughter cells differentiate into memory cells which are easier to activate and enable rapid secondary immune responses upon re-exposure to the same antigen.

Source: Infection and Immunity, Fourth Edition by John Playfair and Gregory Bancroft (2013). By permission of Oxford University Press. © John Playfair and Gregory Bancroft.

Activation of the adaptive immune system

- Individuals are estimated to have up to 10^{12} different BCR and $10^{16}-10^{18}$ different TCR. This is referred to as your 'repertoire'.
- Each lymphocyte bears a single type of receptor with a unique specificity.
- Interaction between this receptor and a molecule capable of binding it with high affinity leads to lymphocyte activation.
- Lymphocyte activation leads to **clonal** expansion so many daughter cells with identical specificity are produced.
- Clonal proliferation is followed by differentiation of specific lymphocytes.
- Lymphocyte receptors specific for self should be deleted at an early stage of their development.

Revision tip

Do not confuse somatic recombination followed by positive/negative selection with clonal selection. Somatic recombination is the random rearrangement of TCR and BCR. Positive and negative selection are checkpoints to ensure that the rearranged receptors are useful (positive selection) but not dangerous (i.e.bind to self with high affinity, these are deleted by negative selection). This is part of lymphocyte maturation and takes place in primary lymphoid organs (bone marrow and thymus, see Chapter 1, section 1.5, Structure, cells and mediators of the immune system). In contrast, clonal selection is about the activation of lymphocytes and it takes place in secondary lymphoid organs, e.g. lymph nodes. It takes place during the course of an immune response and leads to the resolution of infection.

Check your understanding

Explain how pathogens are 'sensed' by cells of the innate defences. (*Hint: The answer should include a definition of how pattern recognition receptors (PRR) recognize pathogen-associated molecular patterns (PAMP) and toll-like receptors (TLR). The basic principles of how different signals are transduced by different classes of TLR in response to extracellular pathogens (and intracellular viruses, e.g. endosomal TLR3, 7, 9) should be explained. You should include details of the inflammasome (NLRs: nucleotide binding and oligomerization domain; activation of inflammatory caspases CARD) and RLRs (helicase superfamily, caspase activation domains CARD). A good answer will include specific examples of PRR (e.g. collectins), and TLR plus detail of the signals produced following 'sensing' (NFκβ, etc.) and the activation of new genes, e.g. pro-inflammatory cytokines IL1-β.)*

How can a finite genome cope with an infinite number of pathogens? (*Hint: This question is about the diversity of antigen receptors (BCR, TCR). This can be explained by the principles of somatic recombination (progenitor cells contain multiple*

VJDC gene segments and the role of RAG1 and RAG2 in randomly selecting one gene segment for each unique rearranged antigen receptor). The number of randomly generated receptors and hypermutation during immune responses (BCR only) should be discussed. A good answer will include the implications of receptor diversity on adaptive immune responses (i.e. the need for thymic education and how this enables us to make such diverse immune responses specifically).)

What are the hallmarks of the adaptive immune response? Explain these in the context of the clonal selection hypothesis. (*Hint: The hallmarks of the adaptive immune response are that it is specific, diverse, memory, escalating response, property of lymphocytes. The clonal selection hypothesis should be described and related to each of these (i.e. lymphocytes express unique preformed receptors, antigen encounter selects cells for activation, proliferation and differentiation, expanded populations of memory cells are easier to activate, etc.). A good answer will mention the need for tolerance (central, peripheral) to avoid autoimmunity and how the theory could be disproved (if a single lymphocyte has multiple specificities).*)

McFarlane Burnett defined the clonal selection hypothesis. Give a detailed description of this hypothesis and explain its importance in the activation of adaptive immune responses. (*Hint: This answer should accurately explain clonal selection (preformed receptors, lymphocyte activation, clonal expansion and differentiation) and relate this to the qualities of the adaptive immune response (i.e. diversity, specificity, memory and escalating response).*)

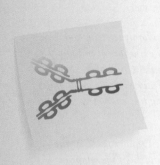

3 How Does the Immune System Destroy?

The purpose of the immune system is to recognize and destroy things that are dangerous. There are a range of effector mechanisms which enable us to eradicate pathogens and control the growth of tumour cells. The type of mechanism depends on the type of pathogen, and we destroy extracellular and intracellular pathogens in different ways. We have also developed particular mechanisms to deal with larger eukaryotic pathogens, e.g. helminths (parasites).

Key concepts in destruction

- The immune system has to recognize and destroy a diverse range of infectious agents which can infect any part of the body (parasites, helminths, yeasts, bacteria and viruses).
- The immune system has to recognize and destroy any transformed body cell.
- There are innate effector mechanisms to destroy extracellular pathogens:
  - Phagocytosis
  - Complement activation
- There are particular innate effector mechanisms to destroy/expel helminths:
  - Eosinophils/goblet cell hyperplasia
- In order to kill intracellular pathogens or tumour cells, the immune system must destroy the affected body cells.

- There are innate effector mechanisms to destroy intracellular pathogens:
  - Natural Killer (NK) cells can destroy infected/transformed body cells
- The adaptive immune system uses similar effector mechanisms but introduces strategies to make them specific:
  - Extracellular pathogens:
    - Antibody-coated pathogens are destroyed by phagocytosis
    - Antibody-coated pathogens can activate complement
  - Helminths:
    - Specific IgE and eosinophils
  - Intracellular pathogens:
    - NK cells can destroy antibody-coated cells (**antibody-dependent cellular cytotoxicity (ADCC)**)
    - Cytotoxic T lymphocytes (CTL) can destroy infected/transformed body cells

3.1 DESTRUCTION: INNATE EFFECTOR MECHANISMS

There are two main mechanisms for destroying extracellular pathogens: **phagocytosis** and **complement** fixation.

Phagocytosis

- There are two major classes of phagocytes, **macrophages** and **neutrophils**.

Key features of phagocytes

System	Mononuclear phagocyte system	Polymorphonuclear system
Effector	**Monocyte**/macrophage Usually named where they reside: • Kupffer cells in the liver • Alveolar macrophages in the lung • Microglial cells in the brain • Osteoclasts in the bone • Mesangial cells in the kidney • Histiocytes in tissue	Neutrophil Sometimes referred to as a granulocyte or a polymorphonuclear cell (PMN)
Identification (nuclear staining)	Mononuclear	Lobed nucleus
Characteristics	Circulating monocytes have a half-life of 1–2 days, and differentiate into long-lived tissue—resident macrophages.	Most common white blood cell (50–70%). Bone marrow produces 1–2×10^{11} cells/day which are estimated to have a very short half-life (<7h)
Other functions	Secrete pro-inflammatory cytokines Can act as an antigen-presenting cell	Secrete neutrophil elastase Can secrete cytokines (pro- and anti-inflammatory)
	Also function to remove dead cells *(following apoptosis)*	Can also kill by release of extracellular traps (DNA and associated histone proteins), i.e. NETosis

Destruction: innate effector mechanisms

1. Mechanism of phagocytosis

Phagocytosis is a multi-step process (Figure 3.1):

- Membrane binding.
- Uptake into specialized organelles (phagosomes).
- Fusion with **lysosomes.**
- Killing within 'phagolysosomes'.
- Release of microbial products.

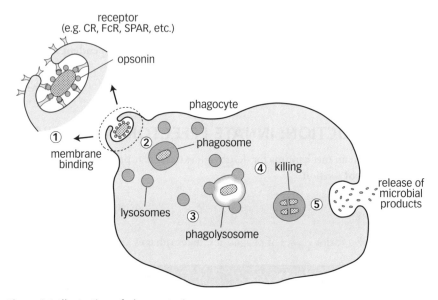

Figure 3.1 Illustration of phagocytosis.

1. Phagocytes internalise pathogens when <u>receptors</u> bind to components on pathogens (e.g. Mannose Receptor binding repeating sugars in the cell wall) or to self-molecules **(opsonins)** bound to the pathogen surface, e.g. C3 coated micro-organisms will bind to complement receptors (CR), antibody-coated pathogens will bind to Fc receptors, organisms coated with surfactant protein A will bind to spA receptors, etc).

2. The bound pathogen is surrounded by the plasma membrane to form an endocytic vesicle called a <u>phagosome</u>.

3. This vesicle acidifies and fuses with <u>lysosomes</u>, granules found in phagocytes which store a large number of acid hydrolases and function to break down protein, lipid and carbohydrate. They also contain anti-microbial peptides and competitors for key substrates needed for pathogen growth (e.g. lactoferrin sequesters Fe^{2+} and vitamin B_{12} binding protein).

4. This produces a large vesicle called a phagolysosome. A multicomponent membrane associated NADPH oxidase is activated by this process and transfers an electron across this membrane leading to a 'respiratory burst' and generation of toxic free radicals.

5. The combined anti-microbial mechanisms are effective at killing pathogens and ultimately microbial products are released from the phagocyte.

2. Killing mechanisms

Lysosomes are granules found in phagocytes which contain a powerful arsenal of anti-bacterial substances. They are delivered to internalized microbes present in the phagosomes via a specialized organelle, the phagolysosome. This is an acidic environment which contains:

- Antimicrobial peptides (e.g. defensins, also known as human antibiotics).
- Proteases, e.g. cathepsin G which damages microbial cells walls and lysosyme which breaks down mucopeptide.
- Glycosidases which break down carbohydrates.
- Sulfatases which degrade sulfur-containing molecules.
- Lipases which break down fats.
- Lactoferrin which binds to free iron (essential for microbial growth).
- Numerous lysosome-associated membrane-bound proteins (LAMPs).

Revision tip

Don't confuse lysosomes with lysozyme—an anti-bacterial enzyme found in tears and saliva which can digest peptidoglycans in bacterial cell walls.

3. Generation of free radicals

In addition, the process of phagocytosis leads to the formation of **reactive oxygen species (ROS)** and **reactive nitrogen species (RNS)** which are also delivered to the phagosome/phagolysosome and contribute significantly to killing of micro-organisms. Your phagocytes can generate free radicals, i.e. their own molecular 'bleach'!

- Phagocytosis stimulates an increase in electron movement across the plasma membrane (increasing redox potential) and ultimately a reduction in molecular oxygen to produce superoxide anion radicals

$$\text{NADPH} + O_2 \xrightarrow{\text{NADPH Oxidase}} \text{NADP}^+ + O_2^{\cdot}$$

- $O_2^{\cdot}$ is a very unstable free radical and breaks down to metabolites including:
  - H_2O_2 (hydrogen peroxide)
  - $^{\cdot}OH$ (hydroxyl radicals)
- Phagocytes also contain an inducible nitric oxide synthase (iNOS2) in their cytoplasm

$$2 \text{ L-arginine} + 3 \text{ NADPH} + 4 O_2 \rightarrow 2 \text{ L-citrulline} + 2 \text{ NO}^{\cdot} + 3 \text{ NADP}^+ + 4 H_2O$$

- Combinations of $O_2^{\cdot}$ and $NO^{\cdot}$ gives rise to a series of free radicals:
  - $^{\cdot}ONOO$
  - $^{\cdot}NOO$
  - $^{\cdot}OH + NO_2$
- Free radicals are extremely toxic to micro-organisms.

Looking for extra marks?

Very few bacteria can survive the 'killing machinery' of our phagocytes. Those that do represent important human pathogens, e.g. *Mycobacteria* spp. which are responsible for tuberculosis and leprosy. *M. tuberculosis* is resistant to killing within the phagolysosome and is thought to escape into the cytosol of the macrophage leading to a persistent intracellular infection which is difficult to eradicate.

Complement

Key features of Complement

- The complement system is a series of plasma proteins (C1–C9) that act together in a cascade to:
  - punch holes in pathogen cell walls (via the formation of the membrane attack complex—a polymer of C5b6789n)
  - promote inflammation and chemoattract other immune cells, e.g. neutrophils, mast cells (via the release of C3a, C4a, C5a peptides)
  - activate other killing mechanisms, e.g. phagocytosis by acting as an opsonin (e.g. C3b) and stimulating oxyburst activity in phagocytes

1. There are three distinct pathways that can lead to the activation of the complement cascade

This is often referred to as 'complement fixation' as complement proteins are fixed onto the pathogen cell walls and disappear from the plasma (Figure 3.2).

1. Alternative pathway: binding of C3b to microbial cell walls.
2. Lectin pathway: binding of Mannan Binding Lectin (MBL, a **collectin**) to microbial cell walls.
3. Classical pathway: binding of specific antibodies to microbial cell walls (see section 3.2, Destruction: adaptive effector mechanisms).

2. Four key things to remember are:

1. All complement proteins exist as inactive precursors until split (e.g. C3 converts to two active parts, C3a and C3b). This generally takes place at the site of inflammation.
2. There are two distinct phases of complement activation:
   a. Amplification—the aim is to coat the microbial surface with as much C3b as possible. Each pathway achieves this in a distinct manner.

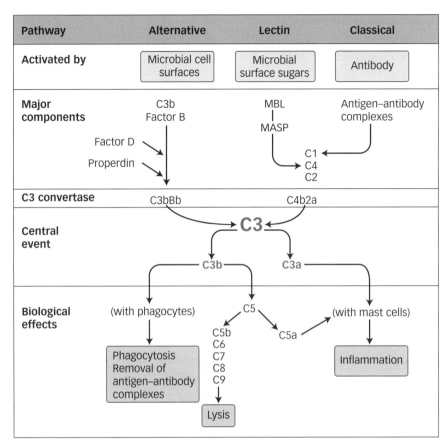

Figure 3.2 Schematic illustration of the complement system. There are three pathways that lead to the activation of the complement cascade (the alternative pathway, the lectin pathway and the classical pathway). There are two distinct stages: (1) The amplification phase which leads to the production of a C3 convertase. This breaks down C3 into C3b which is deposited on bacterial cell surface and C3a, which stimulates inflammation; (2) The lytic phase which leads to the construction of a membrane attack complex (a pore) in the pathogen cell wall and can lead to lysis.

Source: *Infection and Immunity*, Fourth Edition by John Playfair and Gregory Bancroft (2013). By permission of Oxford University Press. © John Playfair and Gregory Bancroft.

    b. Common lytic pathway—the aim is to build a membrane attack complex (a pore in the microbial surface).

3. Complement activation releases bioactive molecules (C3a, C4a, C5a, referred to as **anaphylatoxins**) which stimulate inflammation.

4. Complement-coated microbes are more susceptible to phagocytosis— macrophages and neutrophils express complement receptors (CR) which can bind to C3b (and its derivative iC3b).

Destruction: innate effector mechanisms

3. The alternative pathway

This represents the most ancient pathway, and results when C3b is present in the vicinity of a microbial cell wall.

Stage 1: Amplification
- Serum C3 spontaneously hydrolyses in plasma ('tick over') enabling it to bind to factor B.
- Fluid phase $C3(H_2O)B$ is sensitive to the proteolytic enzyme, factor D.
- This leads to the production of $C3(H_2O)Bb$ which is an active *C3 convertase* that can break down more C3 to form bioactive C3a and C3b.
- C3b is normally rapidly inactivated unless it binds to pathogen cell walls.
- Membrane-bound C3b also binds to factor B (from the serum) to produce a C3bB complex.
- This is split by factor D (serum) to produce more C3bBb (C3 convertase).
- Many more molecules of C3b are deposited on the pathogen cell wall.

Stage 2: Lytic Pathway
- C3 convertase (C3bBb) reacts with more molecules of C3b to generate a complex of C3bBb3b = *C5 convertase*.
- This C5 convertase then splits serum C5 to produce C5b which binds to the complex on the membrane. Bioactive C5a is released.
- C5b binds terminal complement components C6, C7, C8 and C9.
- C9 polymerises to form a pore in the membrane.
- This is the membrane attack complex (C5b6789n).

4. The Lectin Pathway

Mannose-binding lectin (MBL) is an acute-phase protein and a pattern recognition molecule (see Chapter 2, section 2.1). It plays a key role in activating the complement pathway following infection. The ficolin family (also C-type lectins) can also activate this pathway but bind to different targets.

Stage 1: Amplification
- Serum MBL binds to repeating sugars on pathogen cell walls.
- **MBL a**ssociated **s**erine **p**roteases (MASP-1 and -2) are activated and split serum C2 and C4 into 'a' and 'b' components.
- C4b2a complex binds to microbial cell surfaces = *C3 convertase.*
- C4a is released and contributes to the inflammatory response.
- The C3 convertase (C4b2a) cleaves many more molecules of serum C3.
- Many more molecules of C3b are deposited on the pathogen cell wall.

Stage 2: Lytic Pathway
- C3 convertase (C4b2a) reacts with more molecules of C3 to generate a complex of C4b2a3b = *C5 convertase.*

- This C5 convertase then splits serum C5 to produce C5b which binds to the complex on the membrane. Bioactive C5a is released.
- C5b binds terminal complement components C6, C7, C8 and C9.
- C9 polymerizes to form a pore in the membrane.
- This is the membrane attack complex (C5b6789n).

Looking for extra marks?

C3a, C4a and C5a are also known as anaphylatoxins and have multiple biological effects. They stimulate inflammation by increasing vascular permeability, promote **chemotaxis** of phagocytes and mast cells. They can also stimulate mast cell degranulation, which amplifies the inflammatory response. They can also cause smooth muscle contraction. They were identified by their ability to induce a fatal anaphylactic shock when injected into animals.

5. Enhanced Phagocytosis

Pathogens coated with complement proteins are preferentially ingested by phagocytes which express **complement receptors (CR)**.

- Complement receptor 1 (CR1; CD35) is widely expressed by innate effector cells (macrophages, neutrophils, eosinophils) as well as red blood cells, B cells and specialized dendritic cells in lymph nodes.
- CR1 binds to C3b and C4b fixed to pathogen cell walls.
- Phagocytosis is further enhanced by binding with complement receptor 3 (CR3; CD11b/CD18) which can bind to iC3b (a degraded form of C3b on pathogen cell surfaces).

6. Regulation of Complement

The activation of complement is tightly controlled (Figure 3.3 and Table 3.1):

- Complement proteins exist as inactive precursors and work sequentially in a cascade.
- Regulators of complement activation (RCA) and complement control proteins (CCP) block various stages of the pathways.

Looking for extra marks?

Mutations in complement regulatory proteins are implicated in diseases characterized by excessive complement activation. For example, lack of C1-inhibitor is responsible for hereditary angioedema, mutations in Factor H are associated with haemolytic uremic syndrome, age-related macular degeneration, and some forms of glomerulonephritis.

Destruction: innate effector mechanisms

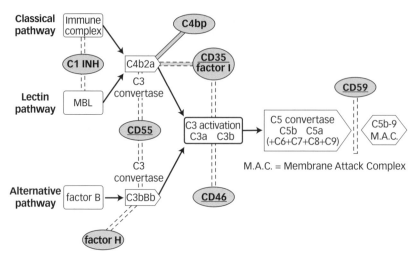

Figure 3.3 Control of complement activation. Membrane-bound inhibitors are underlined.

Name	Action	Inhibits	Features
Factor H	Binds C3b and interferes with C3 convertase C3bBb leading to its decay	Alternative pathway	Fluid phase Synthesized in the liver (hepatocytes)
Factor I	Serine protease that cleaves C3b and C4b blocking the function of C3 and C5 convertases	Alternative, lectin and classical pathways	Fluid phase Synthesized in the liver but can also be made by macrophages, lymphocytes, endothelial cells
C1-inhibitor (serpin peptidase inhibitor)	Forms an irreversible complex with C1r and C1s serine proteases; can bind and inactivate MASP-1 and MASP-2	Lectin and classical pathways	Fluid phase Also inhibits FXIIa, chymotrypsin and kallikrein indicating control of clotting pathways and the generation of kinins
C4 binding protein	Binds to C4b and interferes with C3 convertase C4b2a leading to its decay	Lectin and classical pathways	Fluid phase Also acts as a co-factor for Factor I. Mainly synthesized in the liver (and monocytes)
Decay accelerating factor (DAF) CD55	Interferes with C3 convertase (C3bBb and C4b2a) leading to its decay	Alternative, lectin and classical pathways	Membrane bound Widely expressed (vascular and other tissues)
Complement Receptor 1 (CR1) CD35	Binds C3b and C4b leading to the decay of C3 and C5 convertases	Lectin and classical pathways	Membrane bound Also acts as a co-factor for Factor I. Expressed on leukocytes, red blood cells and in glomeruli (kidney)
Membrane cofactor protein (MCP) CD46	Acts as a co-factor for Factor I mediated cleavage of C3b and C4b	Alternative, lectin and classical pathways	Membrane bound Widely expressed on nucleated cells
CD59 (protectin)	Associates with C9, inhibiting construction of the membrane attach complex (lytic pathway)	Alternative, lectin and classical pathways	Membrane bound Widely expressed

Table 3.1 Key characteristics of Regulators of complement activation and complement control proteins.

Innate mechanisms for destroying intracellular pathogens/ transformed body cells

The only way to eradicate an intracellular pathogen is to destroy the infected body cell. All viral infections are intracellular because they cannot replicate without hijacking the replication machinery of the host cell.

Other pathogens can infect body cells, particularly those which have specific virulence factors enabling them to escape from the phagosome/phagolysosome of phagocytes. These include *Mycobacteria* spp. (which cause tuberculosis and leprosy), *Listeria monocytogenes* (which can cause listeriosis in immunocompromised patients), *Histoplasma capsulatum* yeasts (which cause histoplasmosis), and *Leishmania Major* protozoa which can all survive within phagocytes.

1. Innate immune responses to viruses

The *interferon response* is an essential early protection mechanism against viruses. It 'interferes' with viral replication by up-regulating anti-viral mechanisms in neighbouring non-infected cells (see Chapter 2, section 2.1).

- Viral infection results in the production of a class of cytokines called type 1 interferons (**IFN alpha and beta**) by the infected cell.
- Cytokines (**IFNα and IFNβ**) secreted by the infected cell binds to receptors on neighbouring cells.
- This leads to the activation of second messengers (STAT1, STAT2) and ultimately the transcription of new genes.
- In particular, many interferon-regulated genes (IRG; also referred to as of Interferon-stimulated genes ISG) are activated (more than 2000 have been identified to date).
- These have a wide range of biological functions including:
  - Reduction of viral replication and host cell DNA replication/protein synthesis
  - Production of 'restriction factors' that interfere with the viral life cycle
  - Upregulation of class I MHC and antigen processing
  - Upregulation of pro-inflammatory cytokines and activation of other immune effectors cells

2. Natural killer (NK) cells

Natural killer (NK) cells are stimulated by type I interferons and pro-inflammatory cytokines (including those produced by activated macrophages) and can destroy virally infected cells. They form the second wave of protection against viruses after the interferon response.

Key characteristics of Natural Killer (NK) cells

- Innate lymphoid cells make up approximately 15% of normal peripheral blood mononuclear cells (PBMC) in healthy adults (more in elderly people).

continued

- A large granular lymphoid cell identified by the expression of CD16 and CD56 and the absence of T cell markers (CD3).
- Thought to be important in defence against viruses and immunosurveillance against tumours.

3. Killing mechanisms

NK cells have the ability to destroy body cells and have to be tightly controlled. This is achieved by a three-stage process:

1. Activation.
2. Recognition.
3. Killing.

1. Activation
- Activated by interferons (type I IFN-α, IFN-β and type II IFN-γ), and pro-inflammatory cytokines (e.g. IL-2, IL-12) to become lymphokine-activated killer (LAK) cells.
- Activated NK cells secrete interferon γ which leads to local inflammation and macrophage activation.

2. Recognition
- 2-stage process mediated by:
  - Inhibitory receptors (Don't kill me, I'm 'normal')
  - Activating receptors (Kill me, there is something wrong. . . viral infection/ tumour **transformation**)
- There are two main classes of inhibitory receptors:
  - Type I: C-type lectin proteins (killer lectin-like receptors KLR, e.g. CD94)
  - Type II: Ig superfamily members (e.g. Killer cell Immunoglobulin-like Receptor KIR family molecules)
- ***Key point:*** All NK cells express at least one inhibitory receptor for a self-class I MHC molecule.
- All body cells expressing class I MHC are protected from NK lysis:
  - If an NK cell inhibitory receptor engages with class I MHC on a normal body cell, an inhibitory signal is sent and the NK cell does not kill
  - Viral infection and tumour transformation often leads to a down regulation of class I MHC rendering the target cell susceptible to NK lysis
- There are two main classes of activating receptors:
  - C-type lectin proteins (e.g. NKG2 family including CD69, CD161)
  - Ig superfamily members (e.g. CD2 and related molecules including CD16)
- A subtype of activating receptors are referred to as 'natural cytotoxicity receptors NCRs' (e.g. NKp44, NKp30 and NKp46). It isn't clear what they bind to, but the ligands are thought to be restricted to stressed/transformed body cells.

- To summarize the potential outcomes (Figure 3.4):
  i. Activating Signal → 'abnormal' ligand on self cell (e.g. altered carbohydrate).
  ii. Inhibitory signal over-rides activating signals → MHC recognition/NO LYSIS.
  iii. Loss of inhibitory signal → No MHC recognition in the presence of an activating signal → TARGET CELL LYSIS.

Revision Tip

It is interesting that both NK cells and T cells recognize MHC class I molecules on target cells. If the MHC class I is expressed, it will present intracellular peptides derived from the cytoplasm (e.g. viral peptides in the case of an infection) to cytotoxic T cells. If a virus wants to 'hide' from the immune system and not be recognized/destroyed by T cells, then it may cause MHC class I molecules to be down regulated. This means the target cell loses its inhibitory receptor so NK cells can now kill. Just like the phrase 'heads you win, tails I lose. . . the infected target cell is destroyed both ways (MHC expressed or repressed)!

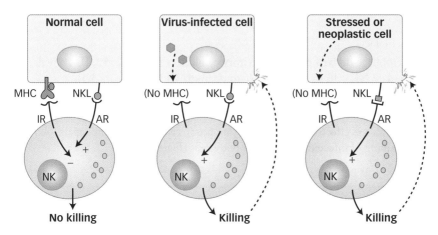

Figure 3.4 NK cells express inhibitory receptors (IR) and activating receptors (AR). Normal body cells are protected from NK cell killing by the inhibitory receptor binding to a self-class I MHC molecule. This inhibitory signal is dominant, and even if an activating receptor can bind to an NK cell ligand (NKL) on a normal cell, no killing takes place. However, *if* class I MHC is down regulated in the case of a viral infected, or neoplastic (transformed)/stressed body cell, then the inhibitory signal is lost. The NK cell will lose the inhibitory signal, and will respond to any NK cell ligand which can bind to its activating receptors resulting in the NK cell killing of the target cell.

Source: Infection and Immunity, Fourth Edition by John Playfair and Gregory Bancroft (2013). By permission of Oxford University Press. © John Playfair and Gregory Bancroft.

3. Killing
- NK cells induce target cells to commit suicide by inducing programmed cell death (**apoptosis**).
- This is a multi-step mechanism involving conjugate formation (between the NK cell and target) and delivery of a lethal hit.
- NK cells induce apoptosis by granule exocytosis:
  - Granules contain **granzymes** and **perforin**
  - They localize to the contact site between the NK cell and target cell
  - Perforin perforates the target cell membrane, granzymes enter the target cell and activate the caspase cascade (cysteine proteases which mediate apoptosis)
- NK cells induce apoptosis by receptor mediated apoptosis:
  - All cells express 'death receptors' (e.g. Fas or CD95, TNFR-I) which express cytoplasmic 'death domains' which can activate the caspase cascade and induce apoptosis
  - NK cells can express Fas ligand (FasL) which binds to Fas, and TNF-related apoptosis-inducing ligand (TRAIL) which binds to TNFR-1. This leads to a conformational change in the cytoplasmic death domains on the target cell (e.g. Fas, TNFR-1) enabling the downstream activators of apoptosis to be recruited

4. Other effects
- Macrophage-derived pro-inflammatory cytokines (TNFα, IL-12, IL-18) will stimulate NK cells to secrete interferon-gamma (IFN-γ) (Figure 3.5).
- IFN-γ will stimulate macrophage activation and further contribute to local inflammation (Figure 3.5).
- Macrophages effectively phagocytose apoptotic cells and promote repair following NK killing of infected/transformed body cells (Figure 3.5).

Revision Tip

Don't forget, NK cells are activated by type I interferons (α and β), they don't necessarily produce them.

Innate mechanisms for destroying Helminths (worms) and parasites

Different effector mechanisms have developed to help us to fight multicellular eukaryotic pathogens which may be too large to phagocytose.

- Damaged epithelial cells at mucosal surfaces produce '**alarmins**' (e.g. IL-25, IL-33, thymic stromal lymphopoietin TSLP) in response to helminth infection.

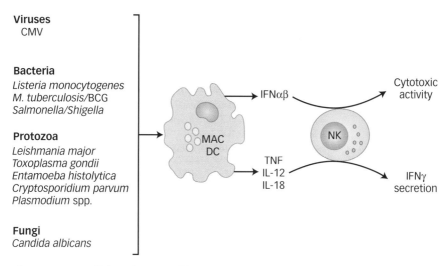

Viruses
CMV

Bacteria
Listeria monocytogenes
M. tuberculosis/BCG
Salmonella/*Shigella*

Protozoa
Leishmania major
Toxoplasma gondii
Entamoeba histolytica
Cryptosporidium parvum
Plasmodium spp.

Fungi
Candida albicans

Figure 3.5 Intracellular infection will lead to the release of type I interferons (α and β) which will activate Natural Killer (NK) cells to destroy infected cells. Macrophage-derived pro-inflammatory cytokines will activate NK cells to produce IFNγ. This will further activate macrophages which play a key role in removing apoptotic target cells and contributing to tissue repair.

Source: *Infection and Immunity*, Fourth Edition by John Playfair and Gregory Bancroft (2013). By permission of Oxford University Press. © John Playfair and Gregory Bancroft.

- Tissue resident **mast cells** act as sentinels to danger. They contain many pre-formed mediators (see Table 3.2) which will stimulate an inflammatory response.
- Tissue resident leukocytes are stimulated to release IL-5 and IL-13.
- This leads to goblet cell hyperplasia which contributes to increased production of mucins/antimicrobial peptides and worm expulsion.
- It also leads to the recruitment of **eosinophils** (eosinophilia) which are directly cytopathic to the parasites.

Cell type	Effector function	Characteristics
Mast cell	Release of vasoactive mediators and pro-inflammatory cytokines	Widely distributed at our epithelial barriers (skin, mucosal membranes). Most inflammatory cells in the body (contains pre-formed TNFα)
Basophil	Release of vasoactive mediators and pro-inflammatory cytokines	Blood borne equivalent of a mast cell
Eosinophil	Release of toxic proteins and cytokines	Blood borne but recruited to tissue in response to appropriate signals

Table 3.2 Innate effectors important in immune responses to parasites.

Destruction: innate effector mechanisms

Family	Characteristic	Mediator
Pre-formed mediators	Biogenic Amines	Histamine, Serotonin (5-HT), Dopamine, Polyamines
	Lysosomal Enzymes	β-hexosaminidase, β-glucuronidase, β-D-galactosidase, Arylsulfatase A, Cathepsins C, B, L, D, and E
	Proteases	Chymase, Tryptase, Carboxypeptidase A, Cathepsin G, Granzyme B, Matrix metalloproteinases, and Renin
	Other Enzymes	Kinogenases, Heparanase, Angiogenin and Active Caspase-3
	Proteoglycans	Serglycin (Heparin and Chondroitin sulfate)
	Cytokines	TNF-α, IL-4, IL-15
	Chemokines	RANTES (CCL5), eotaxin (CCL11), IL-8 (CXCL8), MCP-1 (CCL2), MCP-3 (CCL7), MCP-4
	Growth Factors	TGF-β, bFGF-2, VEGF, NGF, SCF
	Peptides	Corticotropin-Releasing Hormone, Endorphin, Endothelin-1,LL-37/Cathelicidin, Substance P, Vasoactive Intestinal Peptide
	Others	Eosinophil Major Basic Protein (MBP)
Newly formed mediators	Phospolipid Metabolites	Prostaglandins, Leukotrienes, and Platelet Activating Factor
Newly synthesized mediators	Cytokines	IL-33, IL-10, IL-12, IL-17, IL-5, IL-13, IL-1, IL-2, IL-3, IL-4, IL-6, IL-8, IL-9, IL-16, Type I and Type II IFN, TNF-α

Table 3.3 Range of mast cell mediators.

Mast cells and eosinophils contain an impressive array of cytokines and other mediators (Tables 3.3 and 3.4) that stimulate innate immune responses, and can also contribute to the repair process to help resolve tissue damage after inflammation/infection.

Type	Characteristic	Mediator
Pre-formed mediators	Highly basic proteins	Major basic protein (MBP)
	Enzymes	Eosinophil peroxidase (EPO), eosinophil cationic protein (ECP), and eosinophil-derived neurotoxin (EDN) Acid phosphatase, collagenase, arylsulfatase B, histaminase, phospholipase D, catalase, nonspecific esterases, matrix metalloproteinases
	Cytokines	IL-2, IL12, IFNγ, IL-4, IL-13, IL-10, IL-6, TNFα, GMSCF
	Chemokines	IL-8, RANTES (CCL5), eotaxin (CCL11),
	Growth Factors	Stem cell factor
		Transforming growth factor TGFα
		Vitamin B12-binding
Newly formed mediators	Phospolipid Metabolites	Prostaglandins, Leukotrienes, 15-HETE and Platelet Activating Factor
Newly synthesized mediators	Cytokines	IL-1, L-2, IL-3, IL-4, IL-5, IL-6, IL-9, IL-10, IL-11, IL-12, IL-13, IL-16, IL-17, IFNγ, TNFα, GMCSF, TGFα, TGFβ
	Chemokines	IL-8, CXCL1, CXCL5, CXCL9, CXCL10, CXCL11, CCL3, CCL5 and CCL11/eotaxin-1
	Growth factors	Heparin-binding epidermal growth factor-like binding protein (HBEGF-LBP), Nerve growth factor (NGF), Platelet-derived growth factor (PDGF), Stem cell factor (SCF)

Table 3.4 Range of eosinophil mediators.

3.2 DESTRUCTION: ADAPTIVE EFFECTOR MECHANISMS

The adaptive immune response often reuses successful innate mechanisms, but 'adapts' them so they can be activated in a more specific manner.

Antibodies as effector molecules

Antibody-coated targets are rapidly destroyed. Antibodies 'adapt' innate killing mechanisms and improve their specificity and sensitivity so that pathogens are ultimately cleared from the body.

Key characteristics of antibodies

- Antibodies are released by activated B lymphocytes (plasma cells).
- They have an identical specificity to the B cell receptor BCR.
- Antibodies have a common protein structure, i.e. two identical light chains (25kDa; either kappa κ or lambda λ) and two identical heavy chains (50kDa) (Figure 3.6).
- Antibodies have two functional domains, i.e. two identical antigen-binding domains (specific recognition) and one 'Fc' domain (receptor binding = effector function).
- There are five classes of antibodies which are determined by their heavy chain sequence: **IgM**, **IgG**, **IgA**, **IgE**, and **IgD**.
- There are four subclasses of Ig G (IgG1, IgG2, IgG3, IgG4) and two subclasses of IgA (IgA1 and IgA2) in humans.
- IgM and IgA can form multimers which increases the number of antigen binding sites. IgM exists as a pentamer (or hexamer) in plasma. IgA is a dimer in mucosal secretions (not plasma) (Figure 3.6).
- Antibody classes are distributed differently, i.e. IgG is most abundant in serum, tissues and can transfer across the placenta. IgM is found in serum but is too big to easily enter tissue. Secretory IgA predominates at mucosal surfaces, and maybe the most prevalent antibody in the body. IgE is found associated with mast cells close to our barriers (epithelial surfaces, i.e. mucosa and skin).
- Different antibody classes (and subclasses) have specialized properties and functions which reflect differences in their heavy chain sequences.
- Antibodies can be described as '**agglutinating**', '**neutralizing**', '**complement fixing**' based on these different biological properties.
- Receptors to antibody heavy chains (FcR) which mediate these functions are expressed on immune effector cells (e.g. phagocytes, natural killer cells, mast cells).

Destruction: adaptive effector mechanisms

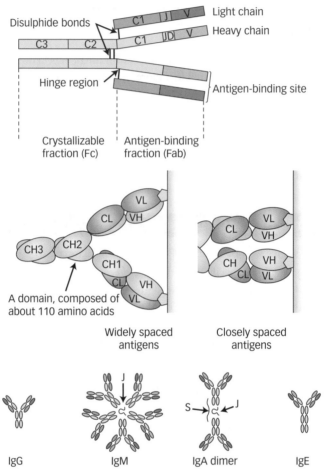

Figure 3.6 The basic protein structure of an antibody (immunoglobulin) molecule. Antibodies are made up of two identical heavy chains and two identical light chains. There are two functional portions: 1. Antigen binding ('Fab' i.e. RECOGNITION) and 2. Biological activity, e.g. complement activation and receptor binding ('Fc', i.e. leading to DESTRUCTION). Each antibody molecule has two identical antigen-binding sites. The protein is organized into Ig domains (each ~110 amino acids). There are constant domains (constant heavy CH domains in the heavy chains and constant light CL domains in the light chains) which contribute to the biological activity. The domains which bind antigen are the variable light (VL) and the variable heavy (VH) chains. The variability arises by the combinatorial diversity of V(D)J recombination and affinity maturation (see text on rearranged lymphocyte receptors in Chapter 2, section 2.2 onwards) so the antibodies have different protein sequences in their variable domains (and therefore three-dimensional structure) which results in different specificities. There are four classes of secreted antibodies, i.e. IgG, IgM (which exists as a pentamer), IgA (which exists as a dimer in mucosal secretions), and IgE. Multimeric antibodies are linked by a joining (J) chain. The differences in heavy chain lead to differences in biological activity of each antibody class. Dimeric IgA binds to the poly-Ig receptor on mucosal epithelial cells which ultimately forms the secretory (S) chain when the complex is secreted.

Source: Infection and Immunity, Fourth Edition by John Playfair and Gregory Bancroft (2013). By permission of Oxford University Press. © John Playfair and Gregory Bancroft.

1. Killing mechanisms

All antibodies have two antigen-binding domains and this determines the specificity of a particular antibody. In addition, each antibody class/subclass will have a different heavy chain or 'Fc' portion. This determines the effector function of the antibody.

The Fc domain can interact with soluble proteins (e.g. C1q) which will activate the complement cascade. Fc domains can also interact with receptors expressed by effector cells, particularly phagocytes and natural killer cells.

'antigen'. They all react with the immunizing antigen, but have different amino acid sequences ('Fab') and recognize different **epitopes**. This is in contrast to monoclonal antibodies (see Chapter 4, section 4.5, Table 4.9) which are a homogenous preparation of antibodies from a single B cell line (hybridoma). They have an identical amino acid sequence and recognize the same epitope. Monoclonal antibodies are very useful tools in research, diagnostics and therapeutics. However, normal immune responses are polyclonal.

2. Activation of Phagocytosis

The dominant antibody in serum is IgG. Phagocytes express Fc receptors for IgG– Fcγ Receptors (Table 3.5). They also express an Fc receptor for monomeric IgA FcαR1.

- Many bacteria can be effectively phagocytosed by macrophages and neutrophils in the absence of antibodies.
- Some pathogenic bacteria possess capsules which help them resist binding and internalization by phagocytes.

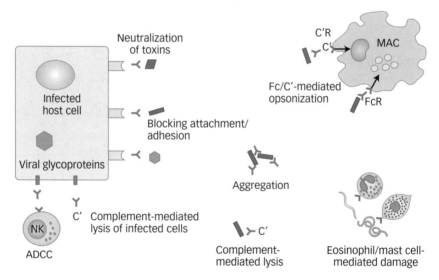

Figure 3.7 A summary of the effector functions of antibodies. Antibody-coated body cells can be targeted for destruction by NK cells and the complement cascade. Antibody-coated pathogens can be destroyed by complement fixation and phagocytosis (two major innate killing pathways for extracellular pathogens). Antibodies can block entry into cells, and neutralize toxins and viruses. IgE antibodies are important in defence against helminths, and specifically harness the inflammatory capacities of eosinophils/mast cells leading to destruction (eosinophils) or tissue changes (e.g. goblet cell hyperplasia) which lead to pathogen expulsion.

Source: Infection and Immunity, Fourth Edition by John Playfair and Gregory Bancroft (2013). By permission of Oxford University Press. © John Playfair and Gregory Bancroft.

Receptor	Expressed by	Binds to	Effect
FcγRI (CD64) High affinity immunoglobulin gamma Fc receptor I	Monocytes and macrophages Can be upregulated on neutrophils during infection	All IgG (except IgG2)	Phagocytosis Antigen capture
FcγRII (CD32) Low affinity Fc receptor (3 isoforms)	Most widely expressed on all myeloid cells (monocytes, macrophages, neutrophils, eosinophils, basophils)	All IgG (including IgG2)	Phagocytosis Clearance of immune complexes
FcγRIII (CD16) Low affinity Fc receptor	Natural Killer cells Some monocytes and neutrophils	IgG	Phagocytosis Antibody-dependent cellular cytotoxicity (ADCC)
FcαR1 (CD89)	Macrophages, neutrophils, eosinophils	IgA (serum)	Phagocytosis Eosinophil activation

Table 3.5 Expression of Fcγ receptors which contribute to phagocytosis.

- Interaction of a specific antibody with a pathogen surface via the antigen-binding domains will lead to a conformational change in the molecule enabling the Fc domains to bind to FcγRs.
- The Fc portion of free antibody does not bind FcγRs.
- This increases the efficiency of internalization and trafficking of pathogens to the toxic phagolysosomal compartment (Figure 3.7).

3. Complement fixation

Certain antibody classes/subclasses will activate the complement cascade upon binding to pathogens. This is known as the classical pathway of complement activation. It is another good example of the adaptive immune system 'adapting' an excellent (but non-specific) killing mechanism by use of specific antibodies (Figure 3.7).

- Antibody bound to its specific target will undergo a conformational change and is called an 'immune complex'.
- The ability of antibody classes/subclasses to activate the classical pathway is: IgM > IgG3 > IgG1 > IgG2 > IgG4.
- IgA and IgE do not activate the classical pathway of complement.

Stage 1: Amplification

- The C1 complex resembles mannose-binding lectin (MBL, which activates the lectin pathway of complement activation). It is made up of a collectin-like molecule (C1q) associated with two serine proteases C1r and C1s.
- C1q can bind directly to pathogen surfaces (pattern recognition), to some acute phase proteins (e.g. C reactive protein, serum amyloid P) or to the Fc domain of bound antibody.
- C1q does not bind to free antibody in solution, and binds preferentially to multiple Fc domains (as would be seen following specific antibody binding to a pathogen surface).

Destruction: adaptive effector mechanisms

- C1r and C1s are activated and split serum C2 and C4 into 'a' and 'b' components.
- C4b2a complex binds to microbial cell surfaces = *C3 convertase*.
- C4a is released and contributes to the inflammatory response.
- The C3 convertase (C4b2a) cleaves many more molecules of serum C3.
- Many more molecules of C3b are deposited on the pathogen cell wall.

Stage 2: Lytic Pathway
- C3 convertase (C4b2a) reacts with more molecules of C3 to generate a complex of C4b2a3b = C5 convertase.
- This C5 convertase then splits serum C5 to produce C5b which binds to the complex on the membrane. Bioactive C5a is released.
- C5b binds terminal complement components C6, C7, C8 and C9.
- C9 polymerizes to form a pore in the membrane.
- This is the membrane attack complex (C5b6789n).

Looking for extra marks?

C3b fixed to pathogen surface by any route will bind Factor B and the alternative pathway will lead to amplification of the response. This is thought to be an important contributor to complement mediated tissue injury.

IgA does not activate complement by the classical pathway but there is evidence that aggregated IgA can activate both the alternative and lectin pathways of complement activation. This may be important for the clearance of immune complexes and can contribute to pathology, e.g. IgA nephropathy, systemic lupus erythematosus (SLE) and poststreptococcal glomerulonephritis.

4. Antibody-Dependent Cellular Cytotoxicity (ADCC)
Natural killer (NK) cells express FcR for IgG (CD16; Table 3.5).

- Virally infected cells may express viral proteins which will bind specific antibodies during the course of an immune response.
- Antibody-coated cells can be bound by NK cells.
- This results in target cell lysis or 'natural' cytotoxicity (Figure 3.8).

5. Activation of effectors specific to helminths
Intestinal helminths are multi-cellular eukaryotic pathogens, often with complex life cycles. They stimulate a strong Th2 immune response (see Chapter 2, section 2.3, Table 2.8), and the activation of IgE-secreting B cells, mast cells, and eosinophils.

Antibodies contribute to the specific eradication of parasites by augmenting the responses of mast cells and eosinophils.

- Mast cells and basophils express FcεR1 which bind with high affinity to IgE (10^{10} M^{-1}).
- IgE will bind to mast cells in tissue/basophils in blood.

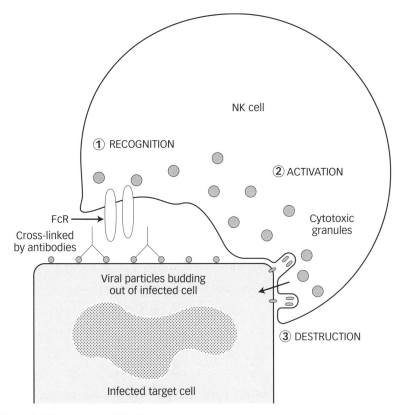

Figure 3.8 Illustration of ADCC.

1. RECOGNITION: Specific antibodies (IgG) bound to viral particles budding out of infected cells (or tumour antigens on transformed body cells) will be cross-linked by the low affinity receptor for IgG (FcγRIII or CD16) expressed on NK cells.

2. This activates the NK cell and causes cytoplasmic granules to move to the contact site with the infected (or transformed) target cell.

3. NK cells kill by granule exocytosis: perforin and granzymes are released from the NK granules and enter the target cell inducing apoptosis or <u>receptor mediated apoptosis</u>: surface expressed fas binds to FasL on the target cell triggering apoptosis *(See section 3.1 Destruction: innate effector mechanisms).*

- Cross-linking of surface bound IgE by specific multivalent antigen will lead to degranulation and release of pro-inflammatory granule contents and synthesize and release lipid mediators of inflammation (Table 3.3).
- Mast cells can also express FcγRs and degranulate in response to cross-linked IgG1.
- Eosinophils express FcγRs, FcεRs and FcαRs, and so can be activated by IgG, IgE and IgA.
- This is often referred to as 'type 2' immunity.

Revision tip

If you are asked how antibodies contribute to killing pathogens, don't forget to stress that their biological function is mediated through their Fc domain (and specificity via their Fab domain). Don't forget to include neutralization, agglutination (IgM), opsonization (IgG and IgA), complement fixation (IgM and IgG), and mast cell (IgE) activation in your answer.

Cytotoxic T lymphocyte (CTL)

Ultimately the only way to recover from a viral infection is to destroy all the virally infected cells. CD8 **cytotoxic T lymphocytes (CTL)** will specifically recognize and destroy virally infected cells. Like NK cells, they have the ability to destroy body cells and have to be tightly controlled. This represents the third wave of the immune response which can lead to the successful eradication of a viral infection (first was the interferon response, then the activation of NK cells). This is achieved by a three stage process:

1. Activation.
2. Recognition.
3. Killing.

1. Activation

- See Figure 3.9.
- CD8 T cells bind to class I MHC/peptide complexes (which are expressed on every nucleated body cell).
- A naive (i.e. not previously activated) CD8 T cell can only be activated by a dendritic cell expressing an appropriate MHC/peptide context in a lymph node (see Chapter 2, section 2.3).
- Signal 1: specific interaction of a particular TCR with a particular MHC-peptide complex on an **antigen-presenting cell (APC).**
- Signal 2: 'non-specific' interaction of CD28 on a T cell with B7 family costimulatory molecules (e.g. CD80/CD86) on an APC. (Note: there are other families of costimulatory molecules that can provide this essential second signal).
- This leads to lymphocyte activation and the production of IL-2 and it's receptor.
- This CD8 T cell now goes through *clonal proliferation* so many identical daughter cells are produced (with the same TCR specificity).
- Additional signals (e.g. IL-2 from a specific CD4 T cell on the same APC) help the CD8 CTL precursor to differentiate into a mature effector cell.

2. Recognition

- See Figure 3.9.
- The activated mature effector CTL will use its T cell receptor and CD8 co-receptor to bind to a specific class I MHC/peptide complex.
- This single signal is sufficient for an activated CTL to kill its target.

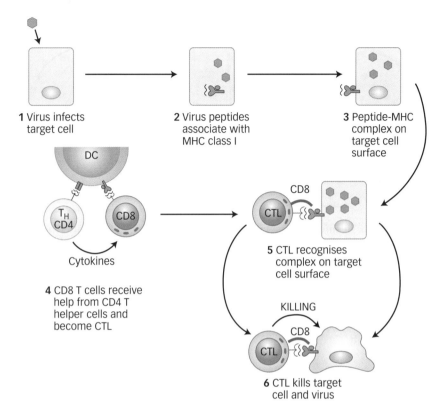

1 Virus infects target cell

2 Virus peptides associate with MHC class I

3 Peptide-MHC complex on target cell surface

DC

T_H CD4

CD8

Cytokines

4 CD8 T cells receive help from CD4 T helper cells and become CTL

CD8

CTL

5 CTL recognises complex on target cell surface

KILLING

CD8

CTL

6 CTL kills target cell and virus

Figure 3.9 Illustration showing how virally infected cells (1) are destroyed by cytotoxic T lymphocytes (CTL). (2) Virally infected cells are sites of viral replication. (3) Viral proteins within the cytoplasm will be processed and presented to newly synthesized class I MHC (see Chapter 2, section 2.3, Antigen presentation). (4) A dendritic cell (APC) will bring viral antigens from tissue into lymph nodes where it will activate specific CD4 and CD8 T cells. A specific CD8 T cell will only differentiate into a CTL if also provided with help (e.g. IL-2) from a specific CD4 helper T cell. (5) The CTL then travels back to the tissue (site of inflammation) and can recognize viral peptides presented by class I MHC specifically. (6) This will lead to destruction of the virally infected target cell.

Source: Infection and Immunity, Fourth Edition by John Playfair and Gregory Bancroft (2013). By permission of Oxford University Press. © John Playfair and Gregory Bancroft.

3. Killing

- See Figure 3.10.
- CTL induce target cells to commit suicide by inducing programmed cell death (apoptosis).
- This is a multi-step mechanism involving conjugate formation (between the CTL and target) and delivery of a lethal hit.
- CTL cells induce apoptosis by granule exocytosis:
  - Granules contain granzymes and perforin
  - They localize to the contact site between the CTL and target cell

Destruction: adaptive effector mechanisms

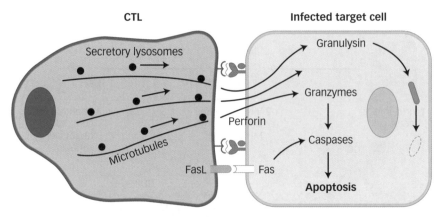

Figure 3.10 CTL kill infected target cells by inducing programmed cell death (apoptosis). If a CTL can specifically bind the class I/MHC peptide complex, then secretory lysosomes are reorganized into the contact site with a target cell. Granzymes and perforin enter the target cell and activate the caspase cascade leading to apoptosis. CTL can also kill by receptor-mediated mechanisms expressing FasL on the cell surface (or in lysosomes) which bind to Fas on the target cell leading to caspase activation and apoptosis.

Source: Infection and Immunity, Fourth Edition by John Playfair and Gregory Bancroft (2013). By permission of Oxford University Press. © John Playfair and Gregory Bancroft.

- ○ Perforin perforates the target cell membrane, granzymes enter the target cell and activate the caspase cascade (cysteine proteases which mediate apoptosis)
- • CTL induce apoptosis by receptor-mediated apoptosis:
  - ○ All cells express 'death receptors' (e.g. Fas or CD95, TNFR-I) which express cytoplasmic 'death domains' which can activate the caspase cascade and induce apoptosis
  - ○ CTL can express Fas ligand (FasL) which binds to Fas, and TNF-related apoptosis-inducing ligand (TRAIL) which binds to TNFR-1. This leads to a conformational change in the cytoplasmic death domains on the target cell (e.g. Fas, TNFR-1) enabling the downstream activators of apoptosis to be recruited

4. Other effects
- • CTL secrete interferon-gamma (IFN-γ).
- • IFN-γ will stimulate macrophage activation and local inflammation.
- • Macrophages will phagocytose apoptotic cells and promote repair following CTL killing of virally infected body cells.

Revision tip

Do not confuse NK cells with cytotoxic T lymphocytes (CTL). Although they may kill by similar mechanisms, they are activated and recognize targets very differently.

Check your understanding

Give a detailed account of the killing mechanisms used by phagocytes. (*Hint: Summarize the multistep mechanism (membrane binding, phagosome/phagolysosome formation) and detail killing by reactive oxygen and nitrogen intermediates plus other lysosomal effects (proteases, defensins, etc.).*)

Give a detailed account of how the complement pathway is activated and controlled. (*Hint: This is asking you to explain the three major routes of complement activation (alternative, lectin and classical pathways) leading to the generation of membrane attack complex. Control of complement should be included (Factor H; DAF; Factor I; CR1; Membrane cofactor 1, CD59).*)

Discuss how Natural Killer cells identify and then destroy virally infected or transformed body cells. (*Hint: The mechanism of NK activation, recognition (inhibitory and activating receptors) and killing (both granule exocytosis and receptor mediated) should be included.*)

Discuss how the immune system deals with viral infections. (*Hint: This is asking you to cover both the innate and adaptive immune responses which are necessary to resolve a viral infection. Innate responses including type 1 interferons and NK cells should be described. The mechanism of NK activation, recognition (including inhibitory and activating receptors) and killing should be included. Adaptive responses by CD8 cytotoxic T lymphocytes (CTL) and resolution of viral infection should be described. CTL activation, recognition and killing should be explained.*)

Antibody molecules are highly variable, effector molecules that play a key role in adaptive immune responses. List the main classes and subclasses of antibodies in humans. How are antibody molecules produced? Explain in detail how antibody diversity develops. (*Hint: The main antibody classes and subclasses are IgM, IgG (1,2,3,4), IgA (1,2), IgE, IgD. Activated B cells differentiate into plasma cells and their B cell receptors (BCR) are released as soluble antibody molecules. A good answer will include T cell help (Th2) and key cytokines (IL4, IL5). You need to include Somatic Recombination (BCR receptor rearrangement) in your answer and summarize the process of VDJC recombination by RAG1/RAG2 during B cell development in the bone marrow to create combinatorial diversity. In addition, Affinity Maturation should include the generation of point mutations during the course of the immune response. Examples of how these are introduced include activation-induced cytidine deaminase (AID) and uracil-DNA glycolase (UNG).*)

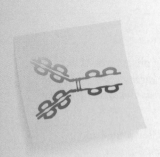

4 The Role of the Immune System in Health and Disease

The immune system plays a key role in keeping you healthy, but it can also contribute to disease under certain circumstances.

Key concepts in health and disease

- A well-functioning immune system should be in balance—it should recognize and destroy those things that cause harm (infectious agents, tumours) but ignore those things which are harmless (normal microbial flora, food eaten, environmental antigens).
- Your lungs, gastrointestinal tract and skin are normally anti-inflammatory environments unless there has been a danger signal/damage which has stimulated inflammation.
- Some individuals have gene defects in immune response genes. These are rare but do help us understand how the immune system works.
- Immunodeficiency can also be caused by external agents (including drugs, radiation and infectious agents). The most common secondary immunodeficiency is caused by a virus (human immunodeficiency virus), but it is not the only cause.
- Immunodeficient patients are more susceptible to infections, do not necessarily respond to vaccines, and may be more at risk of developing tumours.

- Immunodeficiency can also lead to autoimmunity—when the immune system attacks the body.
- Autoimmunity is the breakdown of self-tolerance. Autoimmune diseases are increasingly common (up to 10% of individuals).
- Autoimmunity is mediated by adaptive immune responses (i.e. lymphocytes) and is categorized as organ specific (e.g. type I diabetes) or systemic (e.g. **rheumatoid arthritis**).
- 'Hypersensitivities' are inflammatory immune responses mediated by adaptive immune responses (i.e. lymphocytes). Types I–III are mediated by antibodies (the products of B lymphocytes), and Type IV by cells (T lymphocytes).
- Transplant rejection is also mediated by adaptive immune responses (lymphocytes).
- In contrast, established tumours are anti-inflammatory environments. They show many characteristics which enable tumour cells to escape recognition and destruction. There is evidence that tumours also actively suppress immune responses.
- Immunotherapy aims at inducing adaptive immune responses specific to the tumour. The most successful treatment to date involves blocking two important inhibitors of adaptive immune responses (CTLA-4 and PD-1).

4.1 IMMUNODEFICIENCY

There are two types of immunodeficiency, primary and secondary.

Key features of primary immunodeficiency

- Genetic or developmental defect in the immune system caused by single mutations of immune response genes.
- Present at birth (though may not be detected until later in life).
- Affect either innate or adaptive immune responses.
- Generally very rare (some are X-linked so found mainly in boys).
- Characterized by infections and/or increased risk of tumour development.
- May manifest as an autoimmune disease.
- Can model how the immune system functions.

Key features of secondary immunodeficiency

- Loss of immune function following exposure to various agents, e.g. immunosuppressive drugs, chemotherapeutic agents, radiation.
- Acquired Immunodeficiency Syndrome (AIDS) primarily caused by Human Immunodeficiency Virus (HIV).
- Characterized by repeated infections and an increased risk of tumour development.

Immunodeficiency

Most primary immunodeficiency disorders (PID) are the result of single gene defects. Over 240 different causes have been identified to date.

1. The most common primary immunodeficiency is antibody deficiency

- Poor antibody responses in early childhood (2–3 years).
- Present with upper respiratory tract infections.
- Don't respond to vaccination.
- Immune responses improve at 5–6 years in the majority of cases.
- Treat with prophylactic antibiotics.

2. Common Variable Immunodeficiency (CVID)

- 1–2% of children presenting with antibody deficiencies develop progressively worse antibody responses.
- Low **IgG**, **IgA**, **IgM**. Often have a low lymphocyte count.
- Complex and heterogeneous disorder characterized by increased susceptibility to respiratory and gastrointestinal infections, and complications including autoimmunity, malignancy and granulomas.
- Treated with immunoglobulin replacement therapy (intravenous or subcutaneous).

3. Complement deficiencies

- The complement system is a major effector required to efficiently remove pathogens and focus inflammation at sites of infection.
- Mutations in the complement system have been implicated in a number of PIDs (Table 4.1).
- Low levels of complement proteins can lead to an increased susceptibility to infections.
- However, the inability to control excessive inflammation can also contribute to disease pathology and is linked with autoimmunity and inflammatory diseases.

Disease	Frequency	Complement proteins affected
Systemic lupus erythematosus (SLE)-like, increased infections	rare*	C1q
Rheumatoid diseases (SLE), increased infections	1:10,000–1:20,000 people	C2
Pyogenic infections, atypical haemolytic uremic syndrome (aHUS)	rare	C3
Rheumatoid diseases, SLE-like, increased infections	rare	C4
Meningitis (*Neisseria* spp.), SLE	rare	C5
Susceptibility to infection (*Neisseria* spp.)	rare	C6
Susceptibility to infection (*Neisseria* spp.)	rare	C7
Susceptibility to infection (*Neisseria* spp.)	rare	C8

Susceptibility to infection (*Neisseria* spp.)	rare	C9
Susceptibility to infection (*Neisseria* spp.)	rare	Factor D
Susceptibility to infection (*Neisseria* spp.)/ aHUS	rare	Factor B
aHUS, C3 glomerulopathy (C3G), dense deposit disease, age-related macular degeneration (AMD)	rare	Factor H
aHUS, C3G, AMD, SLE, Rheumatoid arthritis	5% (Caucasians)	Complement Factor H-Related 1
Mild immunodeficiency/recurrent bacterial infections in children	5% (Caucasians)	Mannose-binding lectin (MBL) or its associated serine proteinases (MASP1/2/3)
Hereditary angioedema	1:50,000	C1 inhibitor
Paroxysmal nocturnal hemoglobinuria hemolysis (PNH)	rare	CD46 (MCP)
PNH, chronic haemolysis and relapsing peripheral demyelinating disease cerebral infarction	rare	CD55/DAF
Haemolytic anaemia, polyneuropathy	rare	CD59 (protectin)
SLE	rare	CR1
Infections, SLE, associated with CVID	rare	CR2 (CD21)
Leukocyte adhesion deficiency(LAD), severe bacterial infections	rare	CR3(CD18/CD11b)
LAD, severe bacterial infections	rare	CR4(CD18/CD11c, LFA-1)

*rare: fewer than 200 patients identified

Table 4.1 Complement proteins with gene mutations which can lead to primary immunodeficiency.

4. Phagocyte deficiencies

- Phagocytosis is the other major effector required to clear pathogens.
- Primary immunodeficiency diseases result from either a reduction in neutrophil number (neutropenia $<1 \times 10^9$/l), defective killing capacity (e.g. generation of free radicals), abnormal morphology, defective cell adhesion and migration (Table 4.2).

Defect	*Frequency*	*Effect*
Chronic granulomatous disease	1:250,000 births	Defective respiratory burst. Recurrent infection, granulomas, abcesses caused by *Staphylococcus aureus, Burkholderia cepacia, Aspergillus fumigatus*
Congenital neutropenias	rare	Impaired myeloid differentiation. Severe pyogenic infections, leukaemia
Glucose 6 phosphate dehydrogenase deficiency	rare	Neutropenia, recurrent infection
Myeloperoxidase deficiency	rare	Defective intracellular killing, chronic infection
Chediak–Higashi Syndrome	rare	Impaired migration. Recurrent infection, granulomas
Leukocyte adhesion deficiency	rare	Impaired migration. Severe infections, ulcers, poor wound healing

Table 4.2 Defects in phagocytes which can lead to primary immunodeficiency.

5. Severe combined immunodeficiency (SCID)

These are rare, severe, life-limiting conditions. They are characterized by a lack of functional lymphocytes (T and/or B cells). They present in early childhood with the following symptoms:

- Repeated viral infections from 2–3 months of age, e.g. Respiratory Syncytial Virus.
- Susceptible to bacterial and fungal infections (pneumocystis, candida).
- Constant diarrhoea, failure to thrive, lung failure.
- Need an urgent **bone marrow** (or haematopoietic stem cell) transplant (HSCT).

There are 4 main mechanisms of SCID in humans:

1. Defects in receptor rearrangement, e.g. RAG1/2 deficiency leading to no VDJ recombination of TCR/BCR. No T or B cells (T-B-phenotype).
2. Failure to respond to survival signals, e.g. Common gamma chain deficient leading to defective signals from IL2, IL4, IL7, IL9, IL15 (T-B + NK-phenotype).
3. Defective purine metabolism, e.g. Adenosine deaminase (ADA)/purine nucleoside phosphorylase (PNP) deficiency. Metabolic disorder leading to the build-up of toxic metabolites in T and B cells. (T-B-NK-phenotype).
4. Defects in T cell signalling, e.g. ZAP-70 deficiency leading to an inability to signal through the TCR and results in a selective T cell defect. Selective block of positive selection of CD8+ cells. Leads to a failure of peripheral CD4+ T cell proliferative response. (CD8- phenotype).

Looking for extra marks?

Common gamma chain deficiency (see Chapter 1, Figure 1.9 Common gamma chain cytokine receptor family) is also referred to as X-linked SCID. It has been successfully treated with gene therapy by adding the correct version of the γc gene to a retroviral vector to the patient's stem cells *ex vivo*. T cell reconstitution (in terms of number and function) was observed. However, the retroviral vector preferentially integrated close to an oncogene and 5 of 20 of the first patients developed leukaemia. This remains an experimental treatment, and haematopoietic stem cell transplantation (HSCT) is the standard therapy at present.

---

6. Agammaglobulinaemias

These are severe antibody deficiencies caused by defects in B lymphocytes. They have a similar presentation to SCID and also require a bone marrow transplantation.

X-linked hyper-IgM syndrome
- Defective CD40L.
- No CD40 activation (costimulation, see Chapter 2, Table 2.7) on B cells leads to a failure to class switch.
- **IgM** produced (but not other antibody class, so no **IgG, IgA, IgE**).
- Recurrent bacterial infections (particularly *Pneumocystis Carinii*).

X-linked Agammaglobulinaemia (XLA or Bruton's disease)

- B cell signalling defect characterized by very low levels of IgG.
- Caused by mutations in the gene for Bruton's tyrosine kinase Btk (see Chapter 2, Figure 2.10).
- X-linked (mainly in boys).
- No peripheral B cells.
- Recurrent bacterial infections, particularly otitis, sinusitis and pneumonia, in the first two years of life. The most common organisms are *S. pneumoniae* and *H. influenzae*.

7. Diseases of immune dysregulation

APECED (autoimmune polyendocrinopathy candidiasis ectodermal dystrophy)

- Gene defect of a transcription factor (**auto**immune **re**gulator; AIRE) that causes a rare autosomal disease characterized by a variable combination of organ-specific autoimmune diseases (APECED).
- AIRE controls autoimmunity by regulating the transcription of tissue-restricted antigens in thymic medullary epithelial cells, e.g. insulin.
- The presence of these antigens in the **thymus** allows the deletion of potentially auto-reactive T cells during negative selection (**central tolerance**).
- Failure to express these tissue-restricted antigens in the thymus means that the potentially autoreactive TCR escape into the periphery and can be activated/cause autoimmune disease.

IPEX (Immunedysregulation, polyendocrinopathy, enteropathy, X-linked)

- Gene defect of a transcription factor (FoxP3) which is essential for the development of the Treg phenotype (see Chapter 2, Table 2.8).
- Caused by a failure of regulatory T cell functions.
- Characterized by immunopathology caused by excessive immune activation (severe allergy, haemolytic anaemia, enteropathy, dermatitis, eczema, thrombocytopenia and early death).

ALPs (autoimmune lymphoproliferative syndrome)

- Gene defect in fas (or FasL). Fas-bearing cells are susceptible to cell death following binding to FasL which is expressed by CTL and NK cells.
- Lack of fas expression results in a failure to maintain homeostasis of lymphocyte numbers (by activation-induced cell death) due to defective lymphocyte apoptosis.
- Leads to an accumulation of auto-reactive lymphocytes.
- Characterized by splenomegaly, lymphadenopathy, autoimmune cytopenias, and an increased risk of lymphoma.

8. Auto-inflammatory diseases

These are inherited diseases characterized by prolonged fevers and severe localized inflammation but not associated with autoantibodies. They have been linked with mutations in elements of inflammasome and proteins important in innate immune responses (Table 4.3).

Immunodeficiency

Gene	Expression	Disease
TNFRSF1A (TNF Receptor 1)	Cell surface	Familial Hibernian Fever (or TNF receptor associated periodic syndrome TRAPS)
NLRC4	Cytoplasmic (forms part of an inflammasome complex)	Familial cold auto-inflammatory syndrome
		Auto-inflammation with infantile enterocolitis
NLRP3	Cytoplasmic (forms part of an inflammasome complex)	Familial cold-induced inflammatory syndrome (cold-induced periodic fever, rash, joint pains)
		Muckle–Wells syndrome (periodic fever, rash joint pains, inflammation)
MEFV (pyrin)	Cytoplasmic (forms part of an inflammasome complex)	Familial Mediterranean fever (periodic fever, arthritis)
NOD2	Cytoplasmic (forms part of an inflammasome complex)	Blau syndrome (granulomotus inflammation of skin, eyes and joints)

Table 4.3 Mutations in innate responses which cause auto-inflammatory diseases.

Looking for extra marks?

It is interesting that so many 'fever syndromes' are associated with mutations in the inflammasome complex (see Chapter 2, section 2.1), one of the innate intracellular 'sensors' for pathogens. IL-1β activation is produced following inflammasome activation and a monoclonal antibody specific to this pro-inflammatory cytokine has been approved to treat Muckle–Wells syndrome (Canakinumab, anti-IL-1β).

9. Immune syndromes

These are a group of immunodeficiencies with systemic characteristics. The best characterized are listed below.

DiGeorge's Syndrome
- Most common autosomal dominant defect (1:4000).
- 22q11.2 deletion syndrome.
- Associated with cardiac issues, abnormal facies, thymic aplasia, cleft palate, and hypocalcemia ('CATCH-22').
- Lack (or reduction) of thymic tissue leads to a dysfunction in cellular immune function of varying severity.
- Present with chronic diarrhoea, viral and fungal infections. Susceptible to pneumococcal infections (*Streptococcus Pneumoniae*).
- Antibody deficiencies (failure to make antibodies to polysaccharides).
- Auto-immunity, e.g. Rheumatoid arthritis.
- May benefit from a thymic transplant, bone marrow (or stem cell) transplant or HLA-matched T cell infusion.

Wiskott–Aldrich Syndrome
- Haematopoietic defect (cytoskeleton affected).
- Gene defect mapped to the X chromosome (CD43).

- Cell to cell communication is compromised.
- Present with recurrent bacterial and viral infection, e.g. HSV, EBV and ultimately lymphoma.
- Progressive loss of cellular and humoral immune responses. Increasing severity with age.
- Requires a bone marrow (or stem cell) transplant.

Hyperimmunoglobulin E Syndrome (Buckley–Job Syndrome)
- Characterized by eczema, skin and lung abscesses, hyperextensible joints and recurrent bone fractures, eosinophilia, and high levels of serum IgE.
- Dominant defect in the gene STAT3 (signalling molecule).
- Susceptible to infection, particularly caused by *Staphylococci* spp.

Secondary Immunodeficiency: Human immunodeficiency virus (HIV)

- Human immunodeficiency virus (HIV) is the most common cause of secondary immunodeficiency, but not the only cause. Secondary immunodeficiency is present in any patient taking drugs which affect the bone marrow (e.g. chemotherapy to treat cancer, immunosuppressive drugs to prevent transplant rejection).
- Many pathogens can suppress immune responses, but only HIV will be covered in detail here.
- The World Health Organization (WHO) estimates 35 million people are living with HIV (2013), the majority in sub-Saharan Africa (approximately 25 million) and SE Asia (approximately 5 million).
- WHO estimates that 3.5 million people are living with HIV/Acquired Immunodeficiency Syndrome (AIDS; 2013).
- Caused by an RNA virus (member of the lentivirus family of retroviruses, Figure 4.1) which only contains 9 genes.
- Infects CD4 helper T cells, macrophages and dendritic cells (DC).
- Three phases of infection: acute, chronic, and profound immunosuppression (AIDS).

1. How does HIV infect?
- An envelope protein (gp120) binds to CD4 and a co-receptor (chemokine receptors: either CXCR4 on T cells or CCR5 on macrophages and DC) leading to fusion (with the aid of the other envelope protein, gp41).
- This means some viruses are T cell tropic (and use CXCR4 as a co-receptor) and others are macrophage tropic (and use CCR5 as a co-receptor).
- Nucleocapsid containing viral RNA genome and enzymes enters the cell.
- Viral reverse transcriptase catalyses reverse transcription of ssRNA forming DNA-RNA hybrids.
- RNA template is degraded and second strand of DNA is synthesized to yield HIV dsDNA.
- Viral dsDNA is translocated to the nucleus and integrates into host chromosomal DNA.

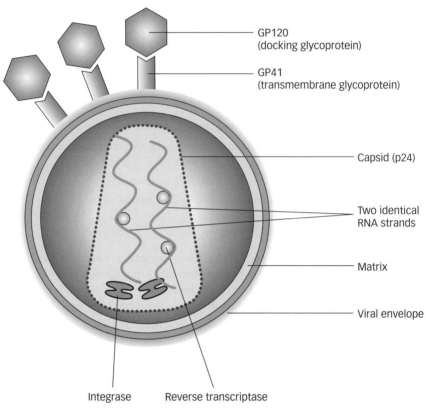

Figure 4.1 Illustration of the human immunodeficiency virus. Two surface expressed envelope proteins are gp120 and gp41. It contains two single-stranded sequences of RNA complexed with reverse transcriptase and integrase enzymes within a nucleocapsid. The virus is highly variable, there are two types, HIV-1 (found worldwide) and HIV-2 (mainly in Africa and India). HIV-1 shows significant genetic variability and is classified into four groups (M, N, O, P) and at least nine subtypes (or clades) of HIV group M are known to exist (A, B, C, D, E, F, G, H, J, K).

Source: A. Hall and C. Yates, *Immunology* (OUP, 2010), 237. By permission of Oxford University Press.

Looking for extra marks?

Genetic variants of chemokine receptors can alter susceptibility to HIV infection. A Δ32 mutation of CCR5 results in a non-functional receptor and is associated with strong protection against M-tropic HIV infection in homozygotes and retarded disease progression for heterozygotes. This mutation has the highest frequency in Northern Russia, Finland, Sweden, Iceland (16%) and Western Europe (10%). Why? There is some evidence that bubonic plague (*Yersinia Pestis*, which wiped out 25–40% of Europeans in the fourteenth and seventeenth centuries) uses CCR5. Other evidence indicates that CCR5Δ32 confers a selective advantage against smallpox.

2. Activation of the pro-virus

- Takes place in activated and not resting T cells.
- Transcription factors stimulate transcription of proviral DNA into genomic ssRNA which becomes processed to mRNA.
- Viral RNA exported to cytoplasm.
- Viral protein production.
- HIV ssRNA and proteins assemble beneath host cell membrane.
- Viral gp41 and gp120 inserted into host membrane.
- Viral particles bud out of host cell.
- HIV has a high replication capacity, e.g. an infected person may produce 10^9 viral particles per day with a half-life of two days!
- HIV replication is error prone and can therefore mutate easily.

3. Acute infection (2–6 weeks)

- Only 20% of HIV infection patients are symptomatic/seek medical assistance.
- 2–3 weeks after infection: sore throat, lymphadenopathy, malaise and joint aches.
- Massive initial increase in viral load (e.g. 1,000,000 copies/ml; acute viraemia) (Figure 4.2).
- Initial decline in CD4 T cells (memory cells).
- Patients are highly infectious and may show some immunodeficiency.

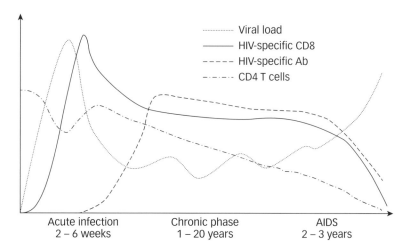

Figure 4.2 Illustration of the three phases of infection with human immunodeficiency virus (HIV). The acquired immunodeficiency syndrome (AIDS) occurs in the later stages of disease.

Source: A. Hall and C. Yates, *Immunology* (OUP, 2010), 241. By permission of Oxford University Press.

4. Chronic phase

- HIV-specific immune responses (antibodies, CTL) develop that can partially control viral replication (Figure 4.2).
- Viral load decreases to 20,000–60,000 copies/ml.
- Lymphoid tissue contains a reservoir of infected macrophages and DC.

5. Symptomatic stage (AIDS)

- Balance between immune response and HIV replication shifts.
- HIV viral load increases (>120,000 copies/ml) (Figure 4.2).
- CD4 T cell count declines below normal limit (500 cells/mm^3).
- When CD4 cells fall below 200 cells/mm^3 there is increased susceptibility to opportunistic infections and certain neoplasms—the patient is immunodeficient.
- Typical infections include: Candida infections, Coccidiomycosis, Cryptosporidiosis, Histoplasmosis, Cytomegalovirus infection, Herpes Simplex Virus infection, recurrent pneumonia and tuberculosis.
- Atypical tumours also develop: Kaposi's sarcoma, non-Hodgkin's lymphoma, invasive cervical carcinoma.

6. Diagnosis of infection

- Presence of anti-HIV antibodies detected by ELISA.
- It takes approximately three months (HIV window) following infection before sero-conversion takes place (although more sensitive tests may detect anti-HIV antibodies within ~3 weeks).
- A positive test needs to be repeated after six weeks.

Looking for extra marks?

ELISA is Enzyme-linked immunosorbent assay. It is a sensitive technique to determine the presence of specific antibodies in a patient's serum or plasma. Viral antigens are coated onto a plastic surface (e.g. a 96-well plate), and if there are any specific antibodies in the serum sample they will bind. Non-specific antibodies are removed by washing (with a detergent solution) and the specific antibody-antigen interactions are detected by addition of a 'conjugate' (anti-human IgG antibodies conjugated with an enzyme). The enzyme conjugated to this secondary antibody will convert a colourless substrate into a coloured product and the intensity can be measured with a spectrophotometer (e.g. a 96-well plate reader). The colour change is directly proportional to the number of antibodies present in the patient. This is called the indirect ELISA and is generally quantified by diluting out the patient's serum, and recording the last positive well. This is known as the antibody titre—the more antibodies present, then the more you can dilute the serum and still see a reaction.

7. Treatment

- HIV cannot be cured but anti-retroviral drugs can inhibit viral replication.
- Highly active anti-retroviral therapy (HAART) can suppress viral load (e.g. <50 copies/ml).
- Anti-retroviral drugs target each stage of the viral life cycle (e.g. fusion inhibitors, reverse transcriptase inhibitors, protease inhibitors, viral integrase inhibitors).
- Viral load and CD4 T cell counts are monitored in HIV patients to evaluate disease progression.
- HIV therapy aims to keep CD4 T cells above 350 cells/mm^3 (>200 cells/mm^3 and immunodeficiency).
- HIV morbidity and mortality rates have fallen in HAART treated patients.
- There are problems with drug toxicity and the development of drug resistant strains.

8. Immune evasion

- It is clear that HIV can mutate during the course of an infection within an individual.
- Patients tend to make oligoclonal T cell responses during the chronic phase of infection (this means only a few clones of different T cells are responding to the virus).
- HIV-specific T cell responses have been shown to exert significant immune pressure on the virus and are driving viral sequence diversity.
- A particular class I MHC (human leukocyte antigens HLA A, B C) will present 9–10 amino acid peptides of HIV, e.g.
  - HLA B27 immunodominant peptide **epitope** is **KR**WIILGLNE (using the 1 letter amino acid code)
  - All peptides that bind HLA B27 have **R** (arginine) at position 2. This is the 'anchor' residue
  - HIV escapes CTL recognition by making a point mutation of this **R** to K (lysine), T (threonine), G (glycine) so that the peptide no longer binds to HLAB27
  - HLA A2 presents the GAGp17 epitope S**L**FNTVAT**L**
  - All peptides that bind HLA A2 have a **L** (leucine) at position 2 and 9 (anchor residues)
  - Single amino acid changes lead to reduced recognition of this immunodominant peptide **epitope**
- Point mutation of HIV at CTL epitopes leads to virus escape.
- This escape leads to an increase in viral load and progression of disease.

9. Vaccination

- HIV mutation and variability is a major problem.
- Different individuals with different HLA will process and present different epitopes of HIV.
- No vaccine is currently effective.

4.2 AUTOIMMUNITY

Autoimmune diseases are adaptive immune responses (i.e. auto-reactive B and T lymphocytes) which cause damage to the patient's own body tissue/cells. Over 80 autoimmune diseases have been described to date (e.g. see Tables 4.4 and 4.5) and their incidence appears to be increasing in populations (estimated up to 10%).

Diseases are characterized into either organ-specific or systemic autoimmune diseases.

Key features of autoimmune diseases

- Complex diseases with varied genetic, environmental and/or pathogenic triggers.
- Varied clinical presentation, multiple disease phenotypes, often relapsing and remitting in their progress.
- Autoimmune diseases are characterized by inflammatory cellular immune responses which are driven by Th1/Th17 helper T cells (sometimes referred to as 'delayed type hypersensitivity' responses).
- Autoantibodies are diagnostic, and may be pathogenic.
- MHC association—certain alleles provide an increased risk for particular autoimmune diseases.
- Difficult to identify disease-specific biomarkers—a single disease has multiple markers, and a single marker is expressed in a number of different diseases.
- Some autoimmune diseases (e.g. SLE) are more prevalent in women (10:1).
- Generally not curable, but may be treatable.

Disease	Source of self antigen	Immunopathology
Addison's disease	Adrenal cells	Autoantibodies
Haemolytic anaemia	Red blood cell membranes	Autoantibodies
Goodpasture's syndrome	Renal and lung basement membrane	Autoantibodies
Graves' disease	Thyroid-stimulating hormone receptor	Autoantibodies
Hashimoto's thyroiditis	Thyroid proteins/cells	Inflammatory T cell and autoantibodies
Type I diabetes (IDDM)	Pancreatic beta cells	Inflammatory T cell and autoantibodies
Myasthenia Gravis	Acetylcholine receptors	Autoantibodies (blocking)
Myocardial infarction	Heart	Autoantibodies
Post-streptococcal glomerulonephritis	Kidney	Antigen-Antibody complexes
Spontaneous infertility	Sperm	Autoantibodies

Table 4.4 Organ-specific autoimmune diseases.

Disease	Source of self antigen	Immunopathology
Ankylosing spondylitis	Vertebrae	Immune complexes
Multiple sclerosis	Brain or white matter	Inflammatory T cells and autoantibodies
Rheumatoid arthritis	Connective tissue, immunoglobulin	Autoantibodies, immune complexes
Scleroderma	Nuclei, heart, lungs, gastrointestinal tract, kidney	Autoantibodies
Sjögren's syndrome	Salivary gland, liver, kidney, thyroid	Autoantibodies
Systemic lupus erythematosus	DNA, nuclear protein, red blood cells, platelet membranes	Autoantibodies, immune complexes

Table 4.5 Systemic autoimmune diseases.

Autoantibodies

Autoantibodies are diagnostic (Table 4.6). They can also contribute to the pathology of the disease.

Autoantibody	Associated Autoimmune disease
Anti-nuclear antibodies (referred to as 'ANA')	Systemic lupus erythematosus, Rheumatoid arthritis, Sjögren's syndrome, Scleroderma, Mixed Connective Tissue Disease
Rheumatic disease serology: 1. Anti-double stranded DNA antibodies (dsDNA) 2. Extractable nuclear antigen antibodies (referred to as 'ENA') 3. Anti-phospholipid antibodies (also known as cardiolipin)	1. Systemic lupus erythematosus 2. Systemic lupus erythematosus, Sjögren's syndrome, Scleroderma, Mixed Connective Tissue Disease, Polymyostis 3. Systemic lupus erythematosus, Anti phospholipid syndrome
Tissue antibodies: 1. Anti-thyroglobulin antibodies (referred to as 'TG') 2. Anti-thyroid peroxidase antibodies (referred to as 'TPO') 3. Anti-gastric parietal Cell antibodies 4. Anti-mitochondrial antibodies 5. Anti-smooth muscle antibodies	1. Hashimoto's Disease, Grave's Disease 2. Hashimoto's Disease, Grave's Disease 3. Autoimmune Pernicious Anemia 4. Primary Biliary Cirrhosis 5. Autoimmune hepatitis
Vasculitis Serology: 1. Anti-neutrophil cytoplasmic antibodies (referred to as ANCA) 2. Anti-myeloperoxidase antibodies (referred to as MPO ANCA) 3. Anti-proteinase 3 antibodies (referred to as PR3 ANCA)	1. Wegener's granulomatosis 2. Wegener's granulomatosis, Vasculitis Associated glomerulonephritis, Microscopic polyangiitis, Eosinophilic granulomatosis with polyangiitis (Churg–Strauss syndrome), Polyarteritis nodosa 3. As 2. above
Rheumatoid arthritis: 1. Anti-cyclic citrullinated Peptide 2. **Rheumatoid Factor (RF)**	1. Rheumatoid arthritis 2. Rheumatoid arthritis, Sjögren's syndrome, some infections

Table 4.6 Common autoantibodies which are used to diagnose autoimmune diseases.

Looking for extra marks?

Motor nerve impulses are transmitted by the release of acetylcholine from nerve endings which bind its specific receptors on the surface of muscle fibres. In Myasthenia gravis, autoantibodies block these acetylcholine receptors thereby preventing signal transmission which leads to muscle weakness.

MHC Associations

Any disease association with MHC indicates that antigen presentation must be involved in the pathogenesis (Table 4.7).

What causes autoimmune diseases?

There is a clear relationship between infection and the development of autoimmune disease. There has been much study of autoimmune populations, the genes they express and the triggers necessary for the development of disease. To summarize:

- Self-reactive lymphocytes exist in healthy individuals.
- In the absence of 'danger' they normally ignore self-tissue.
- Infection stimulates inflammation and causes damage.
- Some pathogen-specific immune responses cross react with self-tissue (**molecular mimicry**) which leads to autoimmune responses (or 'friendly fire').
- Innate responses may also upregulate the immunogenicity of self-peptides, allowing quiescent auto-reactive T and B cells to become stimulated.
- There is a balance between the induction of effector cells to destroy pathogens and regulatory mechanisms designed to limit the immune pathology caused by infection. Autoimmunity may result if this balance is dysregulated.

Disease	Class I MHC	Class II MHC
Addison's disease		HLA DR3
Type I diabetes	HLA A24, B18, B39	HLA DR3, DR4, DQB1
Grave's disease	HLA B08, C07	HLA DR3, DRB1-08
Hashimoto's thyroiditis		HLA DR4, HLA DR3
Myasthenia gravis		HLA DR3
Multiple sclerosis	HLA C05, C15	HLA DR15
Systemic lupus erythematosus		HLA DR3, DR8, DR15
Rheumatoid arthritis		HLA-DRB1, DR4
Ankylosing spondylitis	HLA B27	

Table 4.7 MHC (HLA) associations which predispose to autoimmune diseases

> ### *Looking for extra marks?*
>
> Gram-positive *Streptococcus pyogenes* causes a throat infection and rheumatic fever in children. Antibodies and T cells specific to streptococcal M proteins cross react with heart tissue (cardiac myosin/laminin/tropomyosin). These autoimmune responses are characterized by Th1/Th17 CD4+ T cells and high levels of pro-inflammatory cytokines (TNFα, IL1, IL6, IFNγ). Ultimately the autoimmune response leads to the development of endocarditis and permanent valvular lesions and scarring, so survivors have irregular heartbeats/murmurs for life. Autoimmune complications are more prevalent in individuals with HLA-DR7 and particular variants of the acute phase protein mannan-binding lectin (MBL; 'A' allele is associated with high levels of protein) (see Chapter 3, section 3.1, Figure 3.4).

4.3 HYPERSENSITIVITY

Hypersensitivity is a specific form of the inflammatory response mediated by lymphocytes. The immune response is causing harm and mediating disease pathology. Acute inflammation can be:

1. Local:
   - characterized by redness, swelling (oedema), heat, pain, loss of function
2. Systemic:
   - characterized by fever, sleep and the production of acute phase proteins
3. Hypersensitivity responses:
   - inappropriate specific immunological responses (i.e. mediated by antibodies/ T cells)

Type I hypersensitivity (or immediate type hypersensitivity)

- IgE mediated response to **allergens** (Figure 4.3).
- Allergen-specific IgE binds to its high affinity receptor (FcεR1) on mast cells (also expressed on basophils).
- Cross-linking with the specific allergen causes them to degranulate rapidly.
- This leads to the release of many pro-inflammatory mediators (e.g. histamine, see Chapter 3, Table 3.3).
- Allergic individual experiences vasodilation, smooth muscle contraction:
  - localized anaphylaxis (atopy), e.g. hay fever (allergic rhinitis), asthma, eczema (allergic dermatitis), food allergy (hives or atopic urticarial)
  - systemic anaphylaxis—a potentially fatal allergic reaction, triggered by IgE and resulting in vasodilation (circulatory collapse), smooth muscle contraction (suffocation), pulmonary oedema and loss of consciousness/death if not treated within 30 minutes
- Atopy affects >20% of the population (and the incidence appears to be increasing).

Hypersensitivity

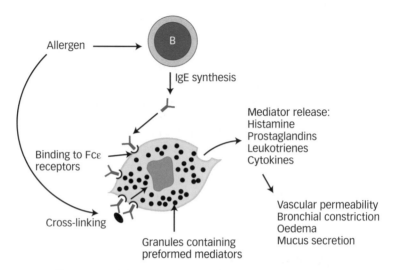

Figure 4.3 An illustration of the development of type I hypersensitivity. An allergen activates an immune response leading to the generation of IgE. This has a very high affinity of FcεR on mast cells (and basophils). Mast cells which bind IgE are referred to as sensitized and will respond immediately when exposed to allergen. Cross-linking will cause immediate degranulation, the release of pro-inflammatory mediators and local or systemic symptoms of inflammation.

Source: Infection and Immunity, Fourth Edition by John Playfair and Gregory Bancroft (2013). By permission of Oxford University Press. © John Playfair and Gregory Bancroft.

- Systemic anaphylaxis affects less than 1% of the population, but the incidence is increasing.
- Common allergens include:
  ○ Pollen (tree, grass), e.g. birch, timothy grass
  ○ Foods, e.g. nuts, seafood, eggs, milk
  ○ Proteins, e.g. foreign serum, vaccines
  ○ Insect products, e.g. bee/wasp/ant venom, house dust mite
  ○ Mold/fungal spores
  ○ Animal hair/dander
  ○ Latex, antibiotics
- Susceptible individuals must first be sensitized (develop a specific IgE response to a particular allergen), allergic responses develop following re-exposure to the same allergen.
- Diagnosis of allergy can be made by injecting the allergen under the skin which stimulates local mast cell degranulation and observation of a 'wheal and flare' reaction within 30 minutes (skin prick test).
- Specific serum IgE antibodies can also be measured.
- Treatment:
  ○ Identify and avoid the allergen

- ○ Immunotherapy (hyposensitization induced by injecting increasing doses of the allergen switches antibody profile from IgE to IgG)
- ○ Anti-histamines—bind to histamine receptors (H1, H2) on target cells
- ○ Adrenalin (to reverse systemic anaphylaxis)
- ○ Anti-inflammatory drugs (corticosteroids)

Looking for extra marks?

Certain individuals have a propensity to make Th2 immune responses and are more likely to develop allergic diseases. This is genetic and certain families will have a higher incidence of hay fever, asthma and atopic dermatitis (it has been estimated that up to one third of Danish and Swedish children are affected by these allergic diseases by the age of five). These atopic individuals make good Th2 responses (IL4, IL5, IL13), have higher levels of IgE and eosinophils.

Type II hypersensitivity

- IgG mediated destruction of antibody-coated cells.
- Activation of cytotoxic cells by antibody-coated cells (e.g. complement fixation, see Chapter 3, Figure 3.7; ADCC, see Chapter 3, Figure 3.8).
- Can lead to blood transfusion reactions and haemolytic anaemias (e.g. of the newborn).
- Antibody-mediated autoimmune diseases (relevant to haematology).

1. Blood transfusion reaction

- Blood must always be cross-matched prior to transfusion to prevent severe transfusion reactions.
- Matching is done to ensure that the recipient does not possess any antibodies that can bind to and destroy the donor blood (Table 4.8).

Genotype	Phenotype	Antigens on rbc	Serum antibodies
AA or AO	A	A	Anti-B
BB or BO	B	B	Anti-A
AB	AB	A and B	None
OO	O	none	Anti-A and Anti-B

Table 4.8 Blood group antigens and corresponding antibodies.

2. Haemolytic disease of the newborn

- This is caused when there is Rhesus incompatibility between mother and foetus.
- Rh– mother/Rh+ baby.
- Sensitization: during birth, the mother is exposed to Rh (foetal blood) and subsequently makes IgG antibodies specific to the Rh+ antigen.

- Re-exposure: in a second pregnancy, maternal anti-Rh+ antibodies will cross the placenta and destroy foetal red blood cells leading to anaemia.
- This is now prevented by screening for Rh− mothers and treating with anti-D antibody (specific to Rh antigen) at birth. This binds to any fetal rbc and destroys them before they can be processed and presented to the mother's immune system.

Type III hypersensitivity

- Caused by immune complexes (generally IgG).
- Arthus reaction—local response following introduction of an antigen. Pronounced erythema (redness) and oedema (swelling) within 4–8 h.
- Mechanism of action is due to excessive antigen–antibody complexes which leads to the activation of complement (see Chapter 3, Figure 3.7).
- This leads to neutrophil chemotaxis and acute inflammation (including lytic enzyme release by neutrophils in the sub-epithelium).
- Inflammatory response causes platelet aggregation, the activation of clotting factors and formation of microthrombi (blood clots).
- Examples include:
  - Serum sickness following addition of large amount of antigen (e.g. 'anti-toxin') leading to fever, rashes, arthritis, kidney damage
  - Autoimmune diseases, e.g. rheumatoid arthritis, systemic lupus erythematosus (SLE), Goodpasture's syndrome show evidence of excessive inflammation due to immune complexes
  - Exacerbates pathological responses during infections, e.g. post-streptococcal glomerulonephritis, meningitis (inflammation of the meninges), hepatitis (inflammation of the liver)
  - Responsible for some drug reactions, e.g. IgG antibodies to penicillin and sulfonamides cause excessive inflammation
  - Responsible for hypersensitivity pneumonitis (extrinsic allergic alveolitis), e.g. farmer's lung caused by immune complexes to inhaled fungi from mouldy compost, hay or corn; pigeon fancier's lung characterized by immune complexes to mucins in pigeon dander
  - Responsible for excessive inflammatory responses to some insect bites

Type IV hypersensitivity (delayed type hypersensitivity)

This is the only hypersensitivity not mediated by antibodies, but by cellular immune responses.

- Excessive cell-mediated immune responses characterized by helper T cells (Th1/Th17), pro-inflammatory cytokines (TNFα, IFNγ), activated macrophages and cytotoxic T cells.
- Typical 'wheal and flare' skin reaction seen after 48–72 h.
- This response is characteristic of transplant rejection and autoimmune diseases.

- Responsible for the formation of granulomas in response to *Mycobacterium tuberculosis*.
- Responsible for contact dermatitis (to metals, e.g. nickel; plants, e.g. poison ivy, poison oak; chemicals, e.g. in cosmetics, hair dyes).

Looking for extra marks?

The mantoux or tuberculin test is done to screen individuals for infection with (or previous exposure to) tuberculosis. Patients are injected in the forearm with 'PPD' (purified protein derivative from *M. tuberculosis*) and then any 'wheal and flare' response determined 2–3 days later. However, it is not specific to infection and can be affected by BCG vaccination/exposure to other *Mycobacterium* Spp.

4.4 TRANSPLANTATION

- Clinical transplantation is an effective treatment for end stage organ failure.
- There are significant benefits in quality of life but patients must take immunosuppressive drugs for the rest of their lives to prevent rejection.
- Kidneys are the most commonly transplanted organs, but hearts, lungs, and livers are other common solid organ transplants.

The types of transplants are defined as:

- Autograft—from one part of the body to another.
- Isograft—between genetically identical twins.
- Allograft—between different members of the same species (clinical transplantation).
- Xenograft—between members of different species.

The laws of transplantation (Figure 4.4):

- Demonstrate that transplant rejection is an adaptive immune response which shows the characteristics of diversity, specificity and memory.

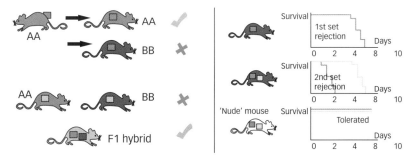

Figure 4.4 Illustration of the laws of transplantation (note: a primary immune response leads to 'first set rejection' and a secondary immune response leads to more rapid 'second set rejection').

Transplantation

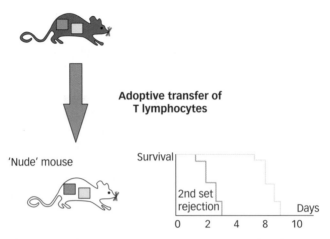

Figure 4.5 *Adoptive transfer experiments demonstrated that T lymphocytes were responsible for the rejection response.*

- Transplants within inbred strains succeed.
- Transplants between inbred strains fail.
- Transplants from an inbred parental strain to an F1 hybrid succeed, but transplants in the reverse direction fail.
- Immunodeficient strains (SCID or 'nude' mouse) can accept any graft.
- It has been shown by adoptive transfer experiments that T cells are essential for graft rejection (Figure 4.5).

Major Histocompatibility Complex

The genetic loci responsible for skin graft rejection was found to be on chromosome 6 and named the 'major histocompatibility complex' or MHC (see Chapter 2, Figures 2.5 and 2.6).

- Class I (HLA A, B, C in humans) and Class II (HLA DR, DP and DQ in humans).
- Peptide receptors.
- Class I MHC bind intracellular peptides/Class II MHC bind extracellular peptides (normally).
- Each MHC molecule can bind 1000s of different peptides.
- Ligands for T cell receptors (thymic selection).
- Most polymorphic gene in the human population genome therefore the chance of having the same genotype as anyone else is extremely low (Figure 4.6).
- MHC molecules are co-dominantly expressed (i.e. both the maternal and paternal allele) therefore each body cell can express up to six different class I MHC molecules i.e. two each of HLA-A, B, and C.
- Class II MHC expression is slightly more complicated. You inherit one copy of HLA-DRα and HLA-DRβ from each parent which can associate to form four different

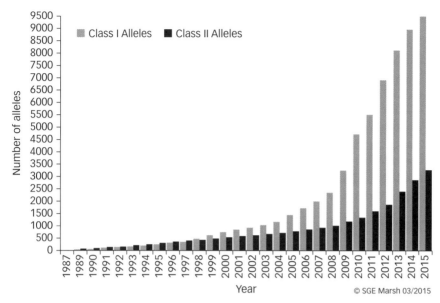

Figure 4.6 Graphical illustration of current known HLA polymorphism.

Source: http://www.ebi.ac.uk/ipd/imgt/hla/intro.html. Reproduced with kind permission of Prof. Steven G. E. Marsh, Anthony Nolan Research Institute, Royal Free Hospital, London.

molecules (i.e. cis forms of maternal alpha with maternal beta chains/paternal alpha with paternal beta chains, plus trans forms, i.e. maternal alpha expressed with a paternal beta chain/paternal alpha chain with a maternal beta chain).

• Therefore antigen-presenting cells may have from 3 to 12 different class II MHC molecules which provides the ability to present a broad spectrum of different peptides from a particular pathogen.

• Differences in MHC alleles mean that different individuals will process and present a different spectrum of peptides from the same pathogen.

• However this also presents a barrier to transplantation as the recipient's T cells can bind to the different donor MHC/peptide complexes.

Revision tip

Don't forget that humans are genetically variable, particularly in immune response genes. Many studies are performed on inbred or identical animals. Human studies are performed on different individuals so there is often a statistically significant variation in how different people respond (although trends may be similar). Imagine a field full of genetically identical sheep (e.g. 'Dolly'), if a pathogen killed one 'Dolly', then every sheep in the field would be susceptible. However, this couldn't happen in the human situation, because we are genetically diverse and we all make different immune responses to the same pathogen. Even if some individuals are susceptible, there will always be other individuals who will be 'resistant'. This gives the species a survival advantage and there will always be survivors to all epidemics and pandemics who pass on their immune response genes.

Direct recognition of donor MHC/peptide complexes by recipient T cells

- T cells from one individual can bind to MHC/peptide complexes from another individual *directly*.
- Affinity for donor MHC/peptide complexes is very high—it has been estimated that up to 10% of all T cells are 'alloreactive', which is a thousand times more than the number of T cells which can bind to any specific MHC-peptide complex during an infection.
- Transplant rejection is an adaptive immune response directed to the allogeneic donor MHC/peptide complexes.
- Clinical transplantation only became possible when immunosuppressive drugs specific to T cells were developed.
- Clinical transplant programmes aim to match the HLA of donors and recipients as far as possible (solid organ transplants generally only determine HLA A, B and DR, however the requirement for matching allogeneic bone marrow transplants is much higher). Identification of HLA on donors and recipients is called 'tissue typing' and is performed by molecular methods (polymerase chain reaction, PCR).
- Better HLA matching is associated with better outcomes (Figure 4.7).

Revision tip

Remember 'allo' comes from the Greek word for 'other' (állos) and is the term used in clinical transplantation to refer to any reaction between genetically different recipients and donors.

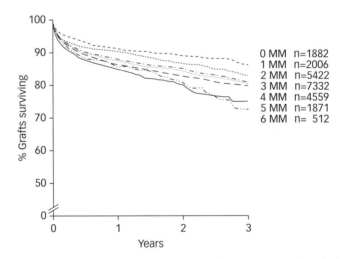

Figure 4.7 Effect of the number of HLA mismatches (MM HLA A, B, DR) on kidney transplant survival. Reprinted from *Transplantation Proceedings*, **33**, Opelz, G., 'New immunosuppressants and HLA matching', 467, Copyright 2001, with permission from Elsevier.

Transplant rejection

The failure of a recipient's body to accept a transplanted tissue or organ is the result of immunological incompatibility (i.e. differences in MHC alleles) and it leads to immune-mediated destruction of the donor organ.

1. Ischaemia/reperfusion injury

- Organ retrieval results in reduced blood flow and oxygenation of tissue.
- Aerobic metabolites are generated.
- Reperfusion leads to the delivery of oxygen.
- The generation of free radicals, e.g. H_2O_2, $OONO^-$, O_2^- which overwhelms anti-oxidant systems.

2. Hyperacute rejection (HAR)

- Rapid—occurs in hours to days.
- Cannot be treated and leads to organ failure.
- Caused by endothelial damage mediated by pre-formed antibodies and complement.
- Rare—can be avoided by ensuring ABO compatibility and the identification of patients with pre-formed antibodies to HLA (donor specific antibodies, DSA).
- Patients become 'sensitized' to HLA by multiple blood transfusions, pregnancy and are more difficult to transplant.

3. Acute rejection (AR)

- Cell-mediated rejection (characterized by Th1/Th17 responses and pro-inflammatory cytokines) and can be referred to as a delayed type hypersensitivity (DTH) reaction (see earlier).
- A variety of effector mechanisms participate in allograft rejection:
  - pro-inflammatory cytokines secreted by CD4+ T cells (e.g. IFN-γ, TNF-α—which upregulate MHC and adhesion expression on the graft cells, IFN-γ promotes macrophage influx and activation leading to tissue damage and IL-2—promotes T cell proliferation and the generation of effector cytotoxic T cells)
  - Direct lysis of class I MHC-bearing cells by CD8+ CTL. CD8 T cells containing perforin are detected during acute rejection episodes and CTL can be isolated from rejecting tissue
  - Antibody-mediated rejection. The development of anti-donor antibodies is associated with complement activation, organ damage and a worse outcome
- Loss of graft function parallels infiltration with mononuclear cells. The number and position of infiltrating mononuclear cells (generally T cells and monocytes) observed in a biopsy from a transplanted organ is used to grade the level of the rejection response.
- Occurs within 10 days and can be reversed by immuno-suppressive drugs.

4. Chronic rejection (CR)

- Aetiology unclear—multiple mechanisms with evidence of Th2 pathology.
- Results in irreversible graft damage (pathological tissue remodelling, fibrosis).
- Occurs in months to years.
- Common, 40% of kidneys lost due to CR.
- No effective treatment.
- Risk factors for chronic rejection:
  - Number and severity of acute rejection episodes
  - Infection (e.g. CMV)
  - Presence of antibodies/plasma cells
  - Complement activation
- CR is the most serious challenge for clinical transplantation.

Looking for extra marks?

The first immunosuppressive drugs which were effective in clinical transplantation were the calcineurin inhibitors (e.g. cyclosporine and tacrolimus). These interfere with the T cell signalling pathway and block T cell activation (see Chapter 2, Figure 2.9). However, care must be taken not to over-immunosuppress and transplant patients are at higher risk of infection and cancer.

4.5 TUMOUR IMMUNITY

Normal body cells have a finite life span, they differentiate and ultimately undergo programmed cell death (apoptosis) and are removed by macrophages. In contrast, a transformed body cell is one which has undergone a mutation which leads to a loss of control of cell division, with the consequence of uncontrolled proliferation.

Key features of tumours

- Tumour cells are healthy body cells and express self/host molecules.
- They seek a blood supply (angiogenesis) to provide the nutrients for growth.
- Malignant tumours metastasize or spread to other sites of the body.
- Established tumours are immunosuppressive environments (characterized by Treg CD4 helper T cells and anti-inflammatory cytokines, e.g. TGFβ and IL10).
- Tumour cells mutate to avoid immune destruction:
  - By avoiding recognition (immune escape), e.g. down regulation of MHC molecules
  - By resisting destruction, e.g. by up regulation of anti-apoptotic molecules
  - By subversion (active immunosuppression), e.g. activation of anti-inflammatory cells and mediators
- The main immune effectors that can destroy tumour cells are NK cells and Cytotoxic T lymphocytes (CTL).

Macrophages are remarkable cells, in addition to their functions of killing pathogens by phagocytosis, stimulating inflammation by cytokine production, and activating memory T cells by antigen-presentation cells (they express class I and class II MHC/peptide complexes), they are also the body's waste disposal system. Apoptotic cells are detected because their plasma membranes flip over, and the phosphatidylserine (PS) (which is usually intracellular) is displayed on the outer surface of the cell. Macrophages express a molecule called Annexin V which can bind to PS with high affinity leading to phagocytosis of the dying/dead cell. This does not lead to inflammation like necrotic cell death.

Do tumours stimulate an immune response?

- Early studies demonstrated that tumours transplanted into mice could be rejected and that this was an immunological response showing specificity and memory.
- Tumours are more common in patients who are immunocompromised, e.g. transplant patients taking immunosuppressive drugs, patients with acquired immunodeficiency syndrome (AIDS).
- Tumour antigens exist and can be recognized by immune effectors (e.g. CTL).
- Malignant progression is accompanied by a profound local immune suppression that interferes with an effective anti-tumour immune response and tumour elimination.
- Vaccination against tumours has therapeutic potential if:
  - A specific immune response to tumour antigens can be induced
  - Long-term memory is induced
  - Vaccines are safe

Tumour antigens

There are many tumour antigens, they can be characterized into two main groups:

1. Tumour-specific antigen (TSA)
- Unique antigen expressed only on the tumour.
- Not expressed by normal cells in the body.
- Unusual.

2. Tumour-associated antigen (TAA)
- Not unique to tumour.
- Antigens normally expressed at very low levels that are expressed in greater quantities in tumour cells.
- Antigens expressed on normal cells during foetal development, not normally expressed in the adult.

Examples of tumour antigens

1. Carcinoembryonic antigen (CEA)

- Expressed by some cancers (especially colorectal, pancreatic, gastric, breast).
- Generally not expressed by normal tissues.
- Decreases with cure and increases with recurrence.

2. HER-2

- **H**uman **E**pidermal Growth Factor **R**eceptor.
- HER-2 proto-oncogene is involved in the regulation of normal growth.
- Gene amplification or HER-2 overexpression stimulates cell growth.
- Occurs in 20–30% of breast cancers.
- Anti-HER2 antibody used diagnostically and therapeutically ('Herceptin').

3. Alphafetoprotein (AFP)

- Markedly increased in most cases of hepatocellular carcinoma (HCC), seminoma.
- May be slightly elevated in benign liver disease.
- Normalizes with response to treatment, increases with recurrence.

Revision tip

Remember, if a tumour antigen is going to stimulate a T cell response, then tumour antigens must be presented by antigen-presenting cells to tumour-specific T cells.

Tumour vaccines

Many different types of 'therapeutic' vaccines have been developed to promote anti-tumour immunity and the destruction of tumour cells. These include:

- Whole tumour cells, peptides derived from tumour cells *in vitro*, or heat shock proteins prepared from autologous tumour cells (undefined tumour antigens).
- Tumour-specific antigen-defined vaccines.
- Vaccines aiming to increase the amount of dendritic cells (DCs) that can initiate a long-lasting T cell response against tumours.

Do they work?

- Antigenic variation is a major problem that therapeutic vaccines against cancer face.
- Tumours have multiple mechanisms of evading immune responses.
- T cell responses are MHC restricted (therefore diverse) which makes tumour antigen selection difficult.

- Therefore to be successful, they need to overcome the low immunogenicity/tolerance which dominates the tumour micro-environment and induce a T cell response, e.g.
  - Combine with existing vaccine (e.g. BCG)
  - Add cytokines to promote antigen presentation (e.g. GMCSF) and T cell activation (e.g. IL-2)
  - Use *ex vivo* generated tumour antigen pulsed dendritic cells/tumour-specific CTL to treat patients
  - Promote costimulation (e.g. anti-CTLA4-Ig antibodies) or block tolerance
- Although some dramatic cures have been seen, this is only in a small minority of patients.

Revision tip

Remember that vaccination is the induction of a specific immune response in order to prevent an infectious disease. However, therapeutic vaccination is the induction of a specific immune response to treat an existing disease.

Looking for extra marks?

Chronic Myeloid Leukaemia (CML) is characterized by the presence of Philadelphia chromosome (an altered chromosome 22 containing a small portion translocated from chromosome 9, i.e. t(9:22)(q34:q11), resulting in the BCR-ABL fusion gene which encodes for a constitutively-activated tyrosine kinase. Detection of the BCR-ABL fusion gene is diagnostic but it is also a target to develop a specific vaccine. Fusion peptide vaccines have been in clinical trials, they have been tolerated well and small numbers of patients have been cured.

Looking for extra marks?

Blockade of negative regulators is proving an effective new anti-cancer treatment. Known as 'checkpoint blockade' immunotherapy, it uses two particular monoclonal antibodies: Ipilimumab = anti-CTLA4 antibodies and Nivolumab = anti-PD-1 antibodies. Combinations are showing 60–80% response rates in metastatic melanoma compared to approximately 10% for single antibody treatment.

Monoclonal antibodies

Monoclonal antibodies play a key role in research and diagnostics (Table 4.9). They are also being used in the treatment of cancer. The number of approved therapeutic antibodies has dramatically increased in the last five years and reflects a change to biological treatment regimes.

Tumour immunity

Trade Name	International Non-proprietary Name (INN)	Target	Type of antibody	Year of FDA approval	Therapeutic indication(s)
Herceptin®	Trastuzumab	HER-2	Humanized IgG1	1998	Breast cancer, Metastatic gastric/gastroesophageal junction adenocarcinoma
Campath®	Alemtuzumab	CD52	Humanized IgG1	2001	B cell chronic lymphocytic leukemia
Zevalin®	Ibritumomab tiuxetan	CD20	Murine IgG1	2002	Non-Hodgkin's lymphoma
Bexxar®	Tositumomab and iodine 131	CD20	Murine IgG2a	2003	Non-Hodgkin's lymphoma
Avastin®	Bevacizumab	VEGF	Humanized IgG1	2004	Metastatic colorectal cancer, Non-small cell lung cancer (NSLC), Metastatic breast cancer, Renal cancer
Erbitux®	Cetuximab	EGFR	Chimeric IgG1	2004	Head and neck cancer, Colorectal cancer
Proximium®	Catumaxomab	EpCAM	Humanized MAb	2005	Head and neck cancer
Vectibix®	Panitumumab	EGFR	Human IgG2	2006	Metastatic colorectal carcinoma
Arzerra®	Ofatumumab	CD20	Human IgG1	2009	Chronic lymphocytic leukemia
	Brentuximab	CD30	Chimeric IgG1 as ADC (antibody drug conjugate)	2011	Hodgkin lymphoma (HL), Systemic anaplastic large cell lymphoma (ALCL)
Xgeva®	Denosumab	RANKL	Human IgG2	2011	Prevention of SREs in patients with bone metastases from solid tumours
Vervoy®	Ipilimumab	CTLA-4	Human IgG1	2011	Melanoma
Perjeta®	Pertuzumab	HER2	Humanized IgG1	2012	Breast cancer
Gazyva®	Obinutuzumab	CD20	Humanized IgG1	2013	Chronic lymphocytic leukemia (CLL)
Cyramza®	Ramucirumab	VEGFR2	Human IgG1	2014	Gastric cancer
Keytruda®	Pembrolizumab	PD1	Humanized IgG4	2014	Melanoma
Blincyto®	Blinatumomab	CD19 & CD3	Murine bispecific tandem scFv*	2014	Acute lymphoblastic leukaemia
Opdivo®	Nivolumab	PD1	Human IgG4	2014	Melanoma
Unituxin®	Dinutuximab	GD2	Chimeric IgG1	2015	Neuroblastoma

Table 4.9 List of therapeutic antibodies approved to treat tumours (note this is just a selection of approved monoclonal antibodies; there are more available to treat other diseases, including transplant rejection and autoimmunity).

*single-chain variable fragment (scFv; This is a heterodimer of antibody VH and VL domains and not a complete antibody molecule).

Check your understanding

Explain the terms primary and secondary immunodeficiency. (*Hint: Primary—genetic or developmental defect in the immune system which is present at birth (though may not be detected until later) and can affect any part of the innate or adaptive responses. Secondary—loss of immune function following exposure to various agents, e.g. drugs, irradiation, viruses, etc.*)

HIV is the major cause of secondary immunodeficiency. Explain why this is the case and in terms of our immune responses to this pathogen, the different stages of disease, its diagnosis and treatment. (*Hint: A clear explanation of how the virus infects T lymphocyte and macrophage/DCs (CD4/chemokine receptor = CXCR4 T tropic and CCR5 macrophage tropic) and its life cycle. The phases of the disease (acute, chronic, AIDS) should be explained plus the particular features of HIV—high replication and mutation capacity. A good answer will discuss immune escape mutations. Diagnosis by ELISA (for specific antibodies) or western blot (for HIV proteins). HIV RNA can be monitored by PCR. Treatment by HAART and the development of resistance.*)

Explain the principle of 'molecular mimicry' and discuss how it can lead to the development of autoimmunity. (*Hint: Students should be able to explain that TCR-MHC interactions can be low affinity, so T cells activated by a pathogen may then cross react with self antigens on tissue. An inflammatory innate response could activate potentially autoreactive T cells. It should be clear that the genetic predisposition is also influenced by environmental factors and there is generally a trigger.*)

Define allergy and explain how it can be diagnosed. (*Hint: Classical allergy is type I or immediate hypersensitivity. It is mediated by IgE antibodies bound to mast cells (via high affinity FcεR1) in tissues which degranulate rapidly following exposure to allergen. This can cause local and systemic inflammation (anaphylaxis). It is diagnosed by the detection of specific IgE antibodies to a particular allergen in vitro or by seeing an immediate 'wheal and flare' response (within 30 minutes) if allergen is applied to the skin.*)

A 23-year-old woman is expecting her first child. Her paediatrician explains that she is at risk of developing Haemolytic Disease of the Newborn (HDN). Why did her doctor identify this risk? Explain how this disease can develop? Describe how this disease can be effectively prevented. (*Hint: This question relates to type II hypersensitivity. It can occur if a rhesus negative patient has a rhesus positive partner. IgG antibodies to Rhesus antigen will develop in the mother following sensitization by the foetal Rh+ red cells. In a subsequent pregnancy, these will cross the placenta and enter the foetal compartment—leading to haemolysis of the rh+ foetal rbc. Administration of Anti-D antibodies will bind to foetal red cells promoting their destruction by the mother's immune system (rather than sensitization).*)

continued

Give a detailed description of how solid organ transplants are rejected. (*Hint: The answer is looking for you to define each stage, i.e. (1) Ischaemia—caused by interruption in the blood supply to the donor organ leading to build up of metabolites followed by oxygen delivery and the generation of free radicals which overwhelms the anti-oxidant system (damage/inflammation). Unavoidable to some extent. (2) Hyperacute—preformed antibodies (complement-mediated destruction, neutrophil recruitment leading to failure to vascularize). Rapid and avoided by screening. (3) Acute—cell-mediated (Th1/Th17) loss of graft function parallels infiltration by mononuclear cells (DTH response). Characterized by pro-inflammatory cytokines, generation of effectors (many mechanisms), generally occurs in the first few months and is reversible with immunosuppressive drugs. Direct recognition of donor MHC/peptide complexes by recipient TCR. (4) Chronic—pathological tissue remodelling (risk—infection and no. of acute rejection episodes), occurs months to years and irreversible.*)

Review the mechanisms by which tumours evade recognition by the immune response. (*Hint: Explain that to destroy a tumour cell then a specific CTL will be needed. Therefore tumour antigens must be presented by APC and activate T cell responses. Define immune evasion strategies (failure to recognize and destroy, ineffective immune responses, sabotage). Examples include failure of effector cells to compete with the growing tumour burden, production of humoral factors by tumours that block cytotoxicity locally, antigen/MHC loss, T cell dysfunction, induction of T regs.*)

Glossary

Acute phase proteins A group of serum proteins that are rapidly produced by hepatocytes (mainly) in the liver in response to inflammation and infection. They play an essential early role in systemic inflammatory responses. They are induced by pro-inflammatory cytokines (TNF alpha, IL-1 beta, IL-6). Increases in serum concentrations of acute phase proteins is an indicator of an acute phase response and the level of systemic inflammation in the body.

Adaptive immunity Adaptive immune responses are those mediated by lymphocytes (B and T cells) which are characterized by rearranged antigen receptors (BCR, TCR). Important characteristics include: (1) specificity, (2) diversity, (3) memory and (4) escalating responses. Adaptive responses are only found in vertebrates (with a jaw) and are quite distinct from **innate immunity** responses.

Adhesion molecules Cell surface molecules that function to bind cells together. They fall into four main families:

- Selectins
- Ig superfamily
- Integrins
- Cadherins

Affinity maturation Affinity maturation refers to the increase in the affinity of antibodies during the course of a humoral immune response. It is particularly important in secondary and subsequent immunizations.

Agglutination A process that causes molecules to clump together. For example, antibodies can cross-link more than one bacterium or virus causing them to clump together. Agglutination of red blood cells (e.g. when cross matching to determine ABO blood groups) is known as haemagglutination.

Alarmins A class of endogenous molecules that signal tissue and cell damage. They are a type of danger signal that activates innate immune responses and promotes aseptic inflammation.

Allergen A type of antigen (generally harmless environmental antigens including pollen, food, protein, insect products, and some chemicals) which generates a specific IgE antibody response. Exposure to the allergen will cross-link specific IgE antibodies on mast cells leading to local/systemic inflammation.

Anaphylatoxin A substance capable of directly triggering complement components C5a, C3a and C4a. This can lead to anaphylactic shock—an often fatal allergic reaction, triggered by IgE or anaphylatoxin-mediated mast cell degranulation and resulting in vasodilation (circulatory collapse) and smooth muscle contraction (suffocation). This is extremely serious if you are unlucky enough to be allergic to nuts or bee venom; such individuals should carry adrenalin in case of emergency.

Anergy A state of specific hyporesponsiveness induced by incomplete antigen presentation. It results if the T cell antigen receptor (TCR) or B cell antigen receptor (BCR) binds to specific antigen (signal 1) in the absence of costimulation (signal 2) or T cell help (in the case of B cells). Anergic lymphocytes will then not respond to fully competent antigen presentation and are more likely to die. T cell anergy can be overcome by exogenous IL-2.

Antibody-dependent cellular cytotoxicity (ADCC) Killing of antibody-coated target cells by binding with Fc receptors. Most ADCC is mediated by NK cells that have CD16 (FcγRIII) on their surface. NK cells activated by bound antibody use similar methods to CTL to kill.

Glossary

Antibody molecules Plasma proteins that bind specifically to particular molecules known as 'antigens'. Specific antibody molecules are produced in response to immunization with a particular 'antigen'. Each antibody molecule has a unique structure that allows it to bind its specific antigen, but all antibodies have the same overall structure and are known collectively as immunoglobulins

Antigen This is a much over-used word in immunology. It was originally used to describe an agent that can react with antibodies (antigen = *anti*body *gen*erator). Today, it is generally used to refer to a substance which generates an immune response. These are generally organisms which infect us, and can be proteins/carbohydrates or even lipids (most rare).

The term antigen is often used interchangeably with immunogen.

Antigen-presenting cells (APC) Specialized cells of the immune system that function to process and present fragments of protein from 'antigens' to T cells.

They express MHC/peptide complexes on their surface for TCR recognition. In addition, to be effective they must also deliver costimulatory signals—mediated by the B7 family (CD80 and CD86) which activate CD28 on T cells.

Professional antigen-presenting cells include dendritic cells, macrophages and activated B cells.

Antigen receptors B and T lymphocytes possess highly diverse receptors for 'foreign antigen'. In the case of a B lymphocyte, the receptor is a membrane-bound antibody molecule (B cell antigen receptor is often referred to as the BCR). It has two binding sites and can recognize the three-dimensional (tertiary) structure of a pathogen.

The T lymphocyte receptor is quite different (The T cell antigen receptor is commonly called the TCR).

Apoptosis Also known as programmed cell death or cell suicide. The term describes a type of cell death that is tightly controlled and which doesn't normally evoke an inflammatory response because the cell's contents are not released. This type of cell death is widespread in nature and often serves a housekeeping function by removing aging or effete cells at the end of their usefulness. The cell's own enzymatic machinery is involved in the eventual destruction of the cell.

Autocrine Effects are those produced by a cell that are exerted on itself. For example, a soluble mediator produced by a cell binds to a receptor on the same cell and exerts a biological effect.

B cell antigen receptor (BCR) Expressed by B cells and composed of a membrane-bound rearranged immunoglobulin associated with Igα and Igβ molecules which contribute to intracellular signalling and B cell activation. The BCR has two antigen-binding hypervariable regions. Once activated, the differentiated B cell becomes an antibody-secreting plasma cell secreting soluble BCR or antibody molecules.

B lymphocyte (or B cell) B lymphocytes are a subset of lymphocytes defined by their expression of a B cell antigen receptor, which is essentially a membrane-bound immunoglobulin molecule. There is massive diversity in BCR, as a consequence of somatic recombination. A B cell can recognize the tertiary structure of pathogens with its receptor (two identical binding sites). Once activated, many copies of the receptor are secreted in the form of antibodies. Somatic hypermutation continues after activation leading to affinity maturation and an increase in antibody specificity.

They play a key role in adaptive responses by:

- presenting antigen to T lymphocytes.
- differentiating into plasma cells and secreting antibody.

Bone Marrow Bone marrow is a specialized micro-environment found inside bone containing many stem cells and growth factors.

It is the primary site of haematopoiesis (production of red and white blood cells).

All bone marrow-derived cells can by characterized by the expression of CD45.

Cadherins The cadherins are a family of calcium-dependent adhesion molecules found throughout the body. They are particularly important in the nervous system and the mucosa. E-cadherin on epithelial cells binds to e-cadherin on other epithelial cells and stick cells together. This is called homotypic binding, and the resultant structure is like a zip. E-cadherin also interacts with the integrin $\alpha E\beta 7$ to retain lymphocytes at epithelial surfaces.

Central tolerance Describes a state of immunological non-responsiveness to self antigens that were present in the thymus. It is a direct result of negative selection during thymic education—thymocytes with a newly rearranged TCR that binds with too high avidity to thymic dendritic cells are deleted by apoptosis.

Chemokine These are a subfamily of chemotactic cytokines classified by their low molecular weight and ability to bind heparin. Over 30 chemokines and 10 receptors have been described. They are very important in leukocyte recruitment and may also play a role in leukocyte activation. There are two main families of chemokines classified on the position of conserved cysteine residues:

- Alpha chemokines (or CXC): e.g. CXCL8 (IL-8), this family predominantly chemoattracts neutrophils.

- Beta chemokines (or CC): e.g. CCL2 (MCP-1), this family predominantly chemoattracts monocytes and lymphocytes.

Note that some chemokine receptors are used by HIV to gain entrance into CD4+ T cells.

Chemotaxis Chemotaxis can be defined as the increased directional movement of cells in response to a concentration gradient of a chemotactic factor (e.g. chemokines).

For example, neutrophils move towards increased concentrations of CXCL8 (IL-8).

Class I MHC Class I MHC consist of an α chain containing three domains, $\alpha 1$, $\alpha 2$ and $\alpha 3$, non-covalently linked to $\beta 2$ microglobulin. $\alpha 3$ is membrane proximal and consists of an Ig superfamily domain (containing S–S disulfide bonds). The $\alpha 1$ and $\alpha 2$ consist of 2 alpha helices on a beta sheet and produce a prominent groove. Their protein structure is very different to class II MHC, but their three-dimensional structure is remarkably similar.

Class I MHC is expressed on most normal body cells. Humans express three different class I MHC molecules (HLA A, B C) and co-express both alleles (maternal and paternal, i.e. you have six different class I MHC molecules on each cell). MHC are the most polymorphic genes known and many alleles exist in the population.

MHC class I is a peptide receptor and cannot fold in the absence of ~9 amino acid peptide (9-mer) in the $\alpha 1$ and $\alpha 2$ groove. Class I peptides are loaded from cytoplasmic proteins by the following mechanism:

- cytoplasmic proteins are broken down into 9-mer peptides under the action of proteosome (catalytic enzyme).

- peptides are transported into the endoplasmic reticulum by TAP (ATP dependent) transporters.

- newly synthesized a chain is stabilized by binding peptide which can then bind b2 microglobulin.

- the assembled class I MHC/peptide complex is transported to the surface for presentation to a CD8 T cell receptor.

Each class I MHC molecule can bind 1000s of different peptides. In general, each allele can bind a different range of peptides depending on the peptide-binding motif of that particular allele. This means that all bound peptides will have one or two amino acids in common that are 'anchor residues', for example, all peptides bound by HLA A2 have a lysine at positions 2 and 9, but the other residues can be any amino acid.

Class II MHC Class II MHC consists of an $\alpha\beta$ heterodimer. $\alpha 2$ and $\beta 2$ domains are membrane proximal and consists of an Ig superfamily domain (containing S–S disulfide bonds). The $\alpha 1$ and $\beta 1$ consist of two alpha helices on a beta sheet and produce a prominent groove. Their protein structure is very different to class I MHC, but their three-dimensional structure is remarkably similar.

Glossary

Class II MHC is generally expressed on specialized antigen-presenting cells of the body which function to activate naive T cells in response to infection. Class II MHC expression can be upregulated on a wide range of body cells (including endothelial cells, epithelial cells, fibroblasts, etc.) particularly by IFN-γ. However, class II MHC is expressed on a surprising number of normal body cells, particularly epithelial cells in mucosal sites.

Humans have three different class II MHC molecules (HLA DR, DP, DQ) and co-express both maternal and paternal alleles.

MHC class II is a peptide receptor and cannot fold in the absence of ~22 amino acid peptide (22-mer) in the α2 and β2 groove. Class II peptides are loaded from extracellular proteins by the following mechanism:

- extracellular/membrane proteins are taken into the cell in endosomes and undergo proteolysis.
- α and β chains, plus an invariant chain (i) are synthesized in the endoplasmic reticulum.
- three αβ heterodimers fold around three invariant chains and are transported to a late endosome.
- early endosomes (containing 'antigen'—extracellular proteins) fuse with late endosomes (containing class II/invariant chain complexes).
- invariant chain is proteolysed to a smaller fragment ('CLIP') which sits in the α1β1 groove (and can be transported to the cell membrane).
- HLA-DM catalyses the replacement of CLIP with extracellular (potentially antigenic) peptides.
- further trimming of the peptide in the α1β1 groove is thought to occur.
- the assembled class II MHC/peptide complex is transported to the surface for presentation to CD4 T cell receptors.

Each class II MHC molecule can bind 1000s of different peptides. In general each allele can bind a different range of peptides depending on the peptide-binding motif of that particular allele.

Clonal Describes a group of cells derived from a single cell by repeated cell division. For example, one cell can yield 32 daughter cells after five rounds of cell division.

Collectins A family of proteins implicated in innate immunity. They include mannose binding protein (MBP), bovine conglutinin and surfactant proteins A and D. They are all collagenous glycoproteins containing groups of C-type (calcium-dependent) lectins that recognize repeating sugar residues typical of bacterial and yeast cell walls, but not mammalian cell walls.

They have a common sub-unit structure consisting of a triple helical collagen-like stalk, a trimeric α-helical neck region and a globular head region containing three carbohydrate recognition domains (CRD).

MBP and SP-A have a structure similiar to C1q, and resemble a bunch of six tulips—each 'head' having three CRD. In contrast, SP-D and bovine conglutinin have a cruxiform structure.

MBP is known to activate complement by the 'lectin' pathway. The other collectins do not activate complement, but facilitate opsonization and intracellular killing by macrophages and neutrophils.

Complement The complement system is a series of plasma proteins (C1–C9) that act together in a cascade to:

(a) punch holes in pathogen cell walls (via the formation of the membrane attack complex—a polymer of $C5b6789n$)

(b) chemoattract other immune cells, e.g. neutrophils, mast cells (via the release of C3a, C4a, C5a)

(c) activate other killing mechanisms, e.g. by acting as an opsonin (e.g. C3b) to facilitate uptake by macrophages and neutrophils and stimulating their oxyburst activity, stimulating basophil and mast cell degranulation and helping antibody production by B cells.

Complement can be directly activated by bacterial cell walls (the alternative pathway), by lectins (e.g. mannose-binding lectin) or by antibody bound to 'antigen' (the classical pathway). Complement activation is often referred to as complement 'fixation' as complement proteins disappear from the plasma and are 'fixed' into pathogen (or host) cell walls.

Each of the three activation pathways leads to the cleavage of C3 under the action of a C3 convertase into soluble C3a and membrane-bound C3b. This membrane-bound C3b combines with other elements of each pathway to produce a C5 convertase. Once this critical enzyme has been produced, a common lytic pathway follows: C5 is cleaved to soluble C5a and C5b. C5b can bind to C6, C7 in serum and this complex (C5b67) can insert itself through cell membranes. This complex then binds C8 which confers on it the ability to bind multiple C9 molecules, which are inserted into the membrane to produce a pore. This pore is made up of C5b-9n and is referred to as the membrane attack complex (MAC).

Complement receptors (CR) Many of the biological activities of the complement system are mediated by their effects on other cells.

There are six known complement receptors (CR) including:

• CR1 (CD35) is expressed on erythrocytes, neutrophils, monocytes, eosinophils, B lymphocytes, and 10–15% of T lymphocytes. It can bind C3b and C4b and this is thought to make these ligands more susceptible to degradation by the plasma serine protease factor I. It results in accelerated decay of C3 and C5 convertases. It plays an important role in the clearance of immune complexes.

• CR2 (CD21) is expressed on B cells. It can bind C3d, C3dg and iC3b (and also Epstein–Barr Virus). It plays an important part in activating B cells and is a good example of how innate responses costimulate adaptive responses. B cell signalling is 1000 times more effective when CD21 and complement are complexed in the BCR complex.

• CR3 (CD11b/CD18 or αMβ2 integrin) is expressed on granulocytes, monocytes, NK cells and some T and B cells. It can bind iC3b as well as ICAM-1-4.

• CR4 (CD11c/CD18 or αXβ2 integrin) is expressed on monocytes, macrophages, NK cells, granulocytes and some T and B cells. It can bind iC3b, fibrinogen, ICAM-1 and CD23.

• C3a/C4a receptor is expressed on mast cells, basophils and neutrophils. It causes mast cell (and basophil) degranulation and neutrophil chemotaxis and receptor ligation can result in anaphylactic shock.

• C5a receptor (CD88) is expressed on mast cells, basophils, monocytes, dendritic cells and binds C5a. It causes mast cell chemotaxis and degranulation and receptor ligation can lead to anaphylactic shock. It belongs to the seven transmembrane serpentine receptor family (like chemokine receptors).

Costimulation Antigen recognition is insufficient to activate lymphocytes. Costimulation defines the additional signal required for proliferation of antigen-specific lymphocytes.

Antigen recognition is commonly referred to as signal 1 and costimulatory signals referred to as signal 2. Examples of costimulatory molecules are listed below.

• Costimulation of T cells is provided by the B7 family (CD80, CD86) on professional antigen-presenting cells binding to its ligand CD28 on T cells.

• Costimulation of B cells is provided by CD40L on CD4 T helper cells binding to CD40L (CD154) on B.

Glossary

C-reactive protein (CRP) Is an example of an acute phase protein. It binds to the phosphoryl choline portion of certain bacteria and fungi, but not on mammalian cells. It contributes to innate defence mechanisms by opsonization and activating the complement cascade (via C1q binding).

It is measured in clinical laboratories to indicate the presence of an acute phase response. Levels of C-reactive protein increase over 1000-fold during infection, inflammation, myocardial infarcation and rheumatic fever.

It is most commonly determined in children thought to have bacterial meningitis, streptococcal pharyngitis and patients with rheumatoid arthritis.

Cytokines Cytokines are proteins made by one cell that affect the behaviour of other cells. They are soluble mediators and can affect the growth, differentiation and function of other cells. They can be defined as intercellular signalling soluble poly- or glyco-peptides which act at pico- or nanomolar concentrations. Only cells with the appropriate cytokine receptor can respond to a particular cytokine.

Effects tend to be paracrine or autocrine, fewer exhibit endocrine action. Most cytokines are secreted and many are held in a reservoir in the extra-cellular matrix.

Cytotoxic T lymphocytes (CTL) T lymphocytes that can kill other body cells. Most CTL are MHC class I restricted CD8+ T lymphocytes, though CD4+ T cells can kill in some cases. They are particularly important in killing intracellular pathogens, such as viruses.

An activated CTL secretes granules containing perforin and granzymes which punch holes in the cell membrane and cause the target cell to commit suicide (apoptosis). The CTL is a serial killer—it first binds to a target cell then delivers a lethal hit and dissociates. This process can be repeated up to six times in a four-hour period! Clearly a dangerous cell that has to be carefully controlled.

Damage-associated molecular patterns (DAMPs) Molecules associated with cellular stress or trauma stimulate innate immune responses. These are endogenous equivalents of infectious PAMPs and promote aseptic inflammation.

Defensins A family of amphipathic antimicrobial peptides that kill bacteria by inserting themselves into their outer membranes resulting in the formation of holes. Defensins are widely distributed in nature and form part of the defence mechanisms of insects and even plants. They are synthesized by neutrophils and epithelial cells and are important mediators of innate defences.

Dendritic cells Dendritic cells are professional antigen-presenting cells capable of activating naive T lymphocytes—i.e. those that have not been activated before. Their name reflects their dendrite like appearance. Dendritic cells sit in tissue and are experts at antigen uptake—you can imagine them wrapped around epithelial cells at all your external barriers (skin, lungs, gut) 'sucking up' their local environment.

When you are infected, damage is caused by the pathogen and it is thought that a 'danger signal' is generated that activates the dendritic cell and sends it running to the lymph node, together with any bits of pathogen from the local micro-environment.

In the lymph node, the dendritic cell matures—it loses the ability to uptake antigen, but becomes exceptionally good at activating T cells. It now expresses high levels of MHC/peptide and costimulatory molecules. Once specific T and B lymphocytes are activated and clonally expand, adaptive immune responses develop that result in the elimination of the invading pathogen.

Endocrine Endocrine effects are those produced by one cell and exerted on a distant cell following transport through bodily fluids. For example, a soluble mediator produced by one cell is transported to a distant site (e.g. via the blood) and binds to a receptor on a distant cell and exerts a biological effect.

Relatively few cytokines exert an endocrine function (though the pro-inflammatory cytokines IL-1 and TNF-alpha can act as 'endogenous pyrogens' and stimulate the liver to produce acute phase proteins).

In contrast, all hormones can be described as 'endocrine'. Hormones tend to be produced by specialized organs and exert their regulatory effects on distant cells/organs. This is quite different from cytokines—which tend to be produced by many cells throughout the body.

Eosinophil Eosinophils are bone marrow-derived cells that are important in defence against parasites. They are only weakly phagocytic and less efficient than macrophages and neutrophils in this respect. They can release granules which contain major basic protein (MBP; highly cationic) and eosinophil cationic protein (ECP; highly basic) which bind to parasites and damage them. They play an important role in inflammation by their ability to release cytokines.

Epitope This is the part of an antigen that a T cell antigen receptor (TCR) or B cell antigen receptor (BCR) will bind to. In the case of TCR, it is the sequence of peptides that bind to an MHC molecule (peptide receptor) on an antigen-presenting cell. BCR bind to the three-dimensional (or tertiary) structure of a molecule, so will be the area of an antigen (amino acids, carbohydrates or lipids) that binds with high affinity to the complementarity determining regions (CDR) in the BCR (or antibody).

Granzymes Granzymes are serine esterases present in the granules of CTL and NK cells. They induce apoptosis of target cells which they enter through perforin channels.

Helper T cells (Th) Differentiated T lymphocytes that can activate other immune cells via the production of cytokines. Most are MHC class II restricted CD4+ T lymphocytes, though CD8+ T cells can also produce cytokines.

The function of helper T cells is driven by the expression of master transcription factors, but it is increasingly appreciated that they are 'plastic' and can change their phenotype under certain circumstances.

Phenotype	Transcription factor	Cytokines produced
Th1	Tbet	IL2, lymphotoxin, TNFα
Th2	GATA-3	IL4, IL5, IL13
Th9	IRF4	IL9
Th17	RORγT	IL17, IL22
Treg	FOXP3	IL-10, TGFβ

CD4 T helper cells play a pivotal role in co-ordinating immune responses. HIV selectively infects and destroys CD4+ T cells with devastating consequences on the immune system. Approximately 1.5 million people died with HIV in 2013—generally of another infection. This is because HIV-infected individuals are severely immunosuppressed and cannot make an effective immune response against pathogens.

High endothelial venules (HEV) HEV are specialized cuboid endothelial cells found in the capillary venule within lymph nodes and spleen. They act as a gateway for lymphocytes to enter the lymph node. They were originally studied by examining the ability of lymphocytes to bind to frozen sections of lymph node tissue. It has been shown that the majority of lymphocytes only bind to the HEV which constitute a very small proportion of cells in the tissue section.

HEV express high levels of adhesion molecules. In peripheral lymph nodes these include CD34 and Glycam-1. This will bind to l-selectin on naive lymphocytes and traffic them into the lymph node. In mucosal-associated lymphoid tissue (peyers patches) HEV express MadCam-1.

IgA Immunoglobulin (Ig) A describes an antibody isotype with an α heavy chain. This is by far the most common antibody in your body, and it plays a key role in protection at mucosal surfaces.

Like IgG it binds and activates macrophages and polymorphs. It also activates complement but by the alternative and lectin pathway, not the classical.

It is present in the serum at 1.4–4 mg/ml as both monomers and dimers. Its binding to microbes on mucosal surfaces prevents them adhering to body tissues and aids their removal by urine, mucus, gastric contents, etc. The role of monomeric IgA present in the plasma is unknown, but it seems to be able to prevent viruses from entering host cells.

IgA is secreted by the plasma cells as dimers, the two basic units being held together by a J chain. The two basic units on a single IgA molecule have the same antibody specificity and so must have been joined before being released from the cell. On the surface of the plasma cell a secretory component is added to the dimer which aids its endocytosis and secretion out of the body by the epithelial cells. IgA specific receptors on the epithelial cells are involved. These secretory receptors are present on the internal surface of the epithelial cells and bind the IgA. Upon release of the IgA onto the mucosal surface the epithelial cell part of the receptor (the secretory piece) remains associated with the IgA and helps to protect it from intestinal enzymes.

IgD Immunoglobulin (Ig) D describes an antibody isotype with a δ heavy chain. It is present on the surface of specific B-lymphocytes along with IgM. They are thought to act together in controlling the activation of the lymphocyte by acting as antigen receptors. IgD has a particularly long hinge region that makes it very susceptible to proteolytic degradation, which may be important in its controlling role. Its labile nature means it has a short half-life—2.8 days compared to 23 days for IgG.

IgE Immunoglobulin (Ig) E describes an antibody isotype with an ε heavy chain. IgE is present at very low levels (17–450 ng/ml) making it harder to study than the other Ig. The basic unit (monomer) structure is like that of IgM with the hinge region being replace by an additional Cε2 (constant) domain.

They bind to mast cells via a high affinity FcεR1 receptor that binds to positions 301–304 of the Cε2 (constant) domain of the IgE molecule. Binding of antigen to IgE results in degranulation of the mast cell. This results in the release of mediators of the inflammatory or acute immune response, e.g. vasoactive amines, cytokines, chemotaxins, etc.

The function of IgE is therefore to protect exposed surfaces from pathogens that have managed to evade IgA on the external surfaces. In addition to the mast cell receptor-binding site IgE is also capable of binding to a low affinity FcεII receptor on inflammatory cells and B lymphocytes via the Cε3 domain.

Importantly, IgE is also responsible for the symptoms of hay fever and extrinsic asthma by causing an inappropriate and excessive response to non-pathogenic allergens.

IgG Immunoglobulin (Ig) G describes an antibody isotype with a γ heavy chain. There are four subclasses of IgG (IgG1, IgG2, IgG3, IgG4). IgG forms 80% of the total immunoglobulin (Ig) and is present in the body fluids (e.g. blood and extra-vascular fluid) as a monomer. Its concentration in the serum is around 8–16 mg/ml. It is the major Ig produced in a secondary response. Its ability to diffuse out into the extra-vascular fluid, combined with its ability to opsonize macrophages and polymorphs and to activate complement by the classical pathway, make it the main line of defence against microorganisms and their toxins.

Specific receptors for the Fc region of IgG are present on the surface of the cells with which the Ig interacts, e.g. the low affinity receptor FcγRII is found on monocytes, neutrophils, eosinophils, platelets and B cells. The result of binding depends on the effector, e.g. opsonization with neutrophils, thrombosis in the case of platelets, down regulation of responsiveness of B cells helping to control antibody production when levels are high.

IgG is very important in the protection of the newborn as it is the only Ig that can cross the placenta (though IgG2 does not cross the placenta as well as the other IgG subclasses). It is also secreted in the colostrum and is capable of crossing the gut mucosa to maintain protection in the infant. This ability to cross these membranes is due to the binding of the IgG Fc region to an Fcγ receptor. The receptor and IgG are then endocytosed into the intestinal cell wall and translocated across and into the infant.

The different IgG subclasses have different amino acid sequences in their Fc regions that result in their different abilities, e.g. varying ability to cross the placenta, IgG4 blocks IgE binding, IgG3 produces spontaneous aggregates.

IgM Immunoglobulin (Ig) M describes an antibody isotype with a μ heavy chain. It is the predominant antibody produced on initial contact with an antigen (primary immune response) and is the first line defence against bacteraemia. It is a large macromolecule (MW 900k), present in the blood at 0.5–2 mg/ml.

It is a polymer of five basic antibody units each with an extra CH (constant heavy) domain, replacing the hinge region and so making the structure more rigid. The five units are bound together by the constant region with the binding sites facing outwards. The five monomers are held together by a small acidic peptide, the J chain, whose main role is probably to stabilize the sulfydryl groups during synthesis so that they remain available for cross-linking between the subunits. The lack of a J chain in certain species indicates that it is not essential for the formation of pentamers and dimers. The five subunits mean that it can bind 10 haptens at once, though if these are large its valency is more likely to be 5. When in free solution it has a star-shaped appearance but conformational changes when it binds to an antigen mean its appearance is more like that of a crab.

As well as being a very effective agglutinator it is also a potent complement activator—cross-linkage of a single IgM molecule being sufficient to activate the classical pathway.

Ig superfamily The immunoglobulin (Ig) superfamily is a family of molecules (70+) thought to have evolved from one common ancestor. They are characterized by the presence of an immunoglobulin domain. This domain or 'fold' is generally 70–100 amino acids organized into two anti-parallel β pleated sheets, which are stabilized by disulfide bonds. Imagine a piece of A4 paper bent over so that the two ends are above one and other—this constitutes the immunoglobulin fold.

A family of adhesion molecules belong to the Ig superfamily, and include ICAM-1 (intercellular adhesion molecule 1, CD54) and VCAM-1 (vascular cell adhesion molecule).

Immuno-receptor tyrosine-based activation motifs (ITAMs) A consensus sequence (*tyrosineXXleucine/isoleucine(X6-8)tyrosineXXleucine/isoleucine where X denotes any amino acid*) found on the cytoplasmic domain of antigen (and some other) receptors which plays a key role in the generation of intracellular biochemical signalling cascades following receptor engagement that ultimately leads to cellular activation. Found in TCR and BCR signalling domains, and some FcR family members.

Inflammasome A family of cytosolic innate pattern recognition receptors that lead to the upregulation of immune response genes. They recruit inflammatory caspases and typically lead to the production of pro-inflammatory cytokines (particularly IL-1β and IL-18).

Inflammation Inflammation is the response to local injury, trauma (aseptic) or infection (septic) and is characterized by an increase in plasma proteins and leukocytes in a local area which contribute to tissue damage and repair. The five cardinal signs of inflammation are pain (dolor), heat (calor), redness (rubor), swelling (tumor) and loss of function (functio laesa).

There are many soluble mediators of inflammation. These include pro-inflammatory cytokines, e.g. interleukin 1 beta (IL-1β), tumour necrosis factor alpha (TNFα) and IL-6, which mediate systemic inflammation and induce the acute phase response. Other examples include Interferon gamma (IFNγ) which plays an important role in local inflammation including the activation of macrophages and lipid mediators of inflammation (e.g. leukotrienes, prostoglandins, platelet activating factor).

Innate immunity Early phases of an immune response depend on innate immunity which includes a variety of mechanisms to recognize and destroy pathogens. It is present at all times and does not increase following repeated exposure (unlike adaptive immunity). The receptors of the innate immune system do not distinguish between pathogens, but are capable of recognizing the common structural elements on pathogens, e.g. yeast, bacterial and viral cell wall structures. For example, lipopolysaccharide (LPS) has a repeating polysaccharide structure which is not present in eukaryotic cells and is recognized by innate receptors (CD14, LPS binding protein, TLR4-MD2).

Integrin A family of heterodimeric membrane glycoproteins expressed on diverse cell types which function as the major receptors for cell-cell adhesion molecules and extracellular matrix. Many integrins bind the RGD (arginine, glycine, aspartate) sequence present in extracellular matrix and other ligands. They all consist of two non-covalently associated subunits (alpha and beta).

Integrins can exist at different affinity states—and integrin affinity is generally upregulated following cellular activation (e.g. after chemokine receptor signalling). They require divalent cations to function.

Genetic deficiencies of integrins do exist. Leukocyte adhesion deficiency (LAD) is a rare inherited disease in which the key functions of leukocytes are impaired, particularly the migration of neutrophils to sites of inflammation. These people suffer from recurrent bacterial infections.

Integrin family All integrins are composed of two non-covalently associated α and β subunits.

Individual α subunits have been shown to associate with more than one β unit, e.g. α4β1 and α4β7

Integrin	β subunit	Other names	α subunit	Other common name	Ligands
VLA-1	β 1	CD29	α 1	CD49a	Laminin (collagen)
VLA-2		or	α 2	CD49b	Collagen (laminin)
VLA-3		VLAβ	α 3	CD29c	Fibronectin, laminin, collagen
		or			
VLA-4		gpIIa	**α4**	**CD49d**	**VCAM-1 (CD106), fibronectin, thrombospondin**
VLA-5			α 5	CD49e	Fibronectin
VLA-6			α 6	CD49f	Laminin
β 1α 7			α 7		Laminin
β 1α 8			α 8		
β 1α V			α V	CD51	Fibronectin
LFA-1	**β2**	**CD18**	**αL**	**CD11a**	**ICAM-1 (CD54), ICAM-2 (CD102), ICAM-3 (CD50)**
Mac-1			**αM**	**CD11b CR3***	**ICAM-1 (CD54), ICAM-2 (CD102), ICAM-4, iC3b, CD23, Kininogen, Fibrinogen, Factor X**
p150,95			**αX**	**CD11c CR4*** p150,95**	**iC3b, Fibrinogen, ICAM-1 (CD54), CD23 (FcγRII)**
CD41a	β 3	CD61 or gpIIIa	α IIb	CD41	Fibrinogen, Fibronectin, Vitronectin, VonWillebrand factor
β 3α V			α V	CD51	as above + Thrombospondin
β 4α 6	β 4		α 6	CD49f	Laminin
β 5α V	β 5	β x, β s	α V	CD51	Vitronectin, fibronectin
β 6α V	β 6		α V	CD51	Fibronectin
LPAM1	**β7**	**βp**	**α4**	**CD49d**	**VCAM-1 (CD106), MadCam1, Fibronectin**
HML-1			**αe**		**E-cadherin**
β 8α V	β 8		α V	CD51	

Elements in bold are of particular importance for leukocyte adhesion

*CR3 and 4 refer to complement receptor 3 and 4.

Interferon alpha and beta (IFNα and IFNβ) or type I interferon These are potent anti-viral proteins that can be produced by most body cells. They are induced by double-stranded RNA (not normally present in mammalian cells) and pro-inflammatory cytokines (e.g. IL-1β and TNFα).

Interferon gamma (IFNγ) or type II interferon IFNγ is a pro-inflammatory cytokine produced by T cells and NK cells. It modifies the biological response of many cells and exerts multiple effects. IFNγ contributes to macrophage activation and local inflammation.

Interleukin-1 β (IL-1β) IL-1β plays a central role in inflammation and immune responses. It is not expressed during homeostatic conditions but can be induced by virtually any nucleated body cell including monocytes, macrophages, B cells, dendritic cells, endothelial cells, epithelial cells, fibroblasts, etc. It modifies the biological response of many cells and exerts multiple effects. The biological effects of IL-β are broadly similar to TNFα and IL-6. It contributes to innate responses by its pro-inflammatory action and stimulates the acute-phase response (together with TNFα, for which reason it is also referred to as an 'endogenous pyrogen' since it raises body temperature). IL-1 contributes to adaptive responses by stimulating T cells (upregulates IL-2 secretion and IL2r expression), and upregulating MHC and costimulatory molecules on antigen-presenting cells. IL-1 is a differentiation factor for B cells and enhances plasma cell development. IL-1 also stimulates tissue repair at the end of an immune response, e.g. by induction of collagenases, and activation of fibroblasts and smooth muscle.

IL-1β is very tightly controlled. It is produced as an inactive precursor which can be processed intracellularly (by caspase 1) and extracellularly. There are two receptors (IL-1RI and IL-1RII) and an accessory protein (IL-1RAcP). The only functional receptor is IL-1RI complexed with IL-1RAcP. IL-1RII is a decoy receptor, and IL-1RI does not signal in the absence of the accessory protein. Membrane-bound and soluble forms of the receptor exist. In addition, the receptor is inhibited by IL-1 receptor antagonist (IL-1Ra) which can exist in two soluble and one membrane-bound form. IL-1Ra competes with IL-1 for receptor occupancy.

IL-1β is viewed as a signature cytokine for inflammasome activation.

Interestingly, high levels of IL-1Ra and a high IL-1Ra/IL-1 ratio are good clinical indicators in disease. Blockade of the receptor antagonist (IL-1Ra) appears to worsen inflammation.

Interleukins (IL-) Interleukins are a sub-group of cytokines that effect the growth and differentiation of immune and haematopoietic cells. To date, IL-1 to IL-37 have been described. They have wide-ranging effects on immune responses.

Most interleukin receptors fall into one of several receptor families:

- The IL-2 receptor subfamily has a common γ chain which can combine with other chains to bind IL-2, 4, 7, 9 and 15.
- The IL-6 receptor subfamily has a common gp130 subunit which can combine with itself/other chains to bind IL-6 and 11 (plus other cytokines).
- The GM-CSF receptor subfamily has a common β chain which can combine with other chains to bind IL-3 and 5 (in addition to GM-CSF).

Lectin A lectin is a family of proteins which bind specific sugars on glycoproteins and glycolipids. Note: glyco = 'sugar'.

Leukocyte This is the general term for a white blood cell. Leukocytes include lymphocytes (T and B), polymorphonuclear leukocytes (PMN; neutrophils, basophils and eosinophils) and monocytes (precursors of macrophages).

LPS LPS stands for lipopolysaccharide. It is an endotoxin derived from gram-negative bacterial cell walls which has inflammatory and mitogenic actions.

Lymph Node Lymph nodes are secondary lymphoid organs where adaptive immune responses are initiated. They are linked together by a system of lymphatics. Their key role is to bring together antigen from pathogens (e.g. brought from tissue by antigen-presenting cells via the lymphatics) and lymphocytes—the key players in adaptive immune responses.

Glossary

The outer region of the tissue is the cortex, which is organized into lymphoid follicles containing B cells and paracortical areas containing T cells. During immune responses, T cells move into the follicles and a germinal centre develops. This becomes an area of massive B cell proliferation. The inner region of the lymph node is called the medulla and contains strings of macrophages and antibody-secreting plasma cells (medullary cords). T cells travel around the body in the blood and enter through specialized **'high endothelial venules'**. They then spend the next 18 hours looking around the lymph node to see if their TCR can specifically recognize any MHC/peptide combinations on antigen-presenting cells. If a TCR is useful, and recognizes a bit of pathogen that has come from tissue (probably on a dendritic cell), clonal selection and adaptive immune responses follow. If not, that T cell leaves the lymph node and moves onto the next lymph node around the body.

A consequence of diversity is that there will be relatively few lymphocytes that can respond to a specific pathogen (estimated to be about 1 in 10,000–100,000). The specialized micro-environment of the lymph node enables these relatively rare pre-formed lymphocyte receptors to come into contact with their specific antigen and adaptive immune responses to take place.

Lymphocyte This term includes B and T lymphocytes (or cells). They are bone marrow derived and are responsible for adaptive immune responses. Their key feature is possession of rearranged antigen receptors—the **BCR** and **TCR**.

Lymphoid diversity B cell receptors (BCR) and T cell receptors (TCR) are highly variable as a result of genetic rearrangement of multiple exons (V, D, J) of germline DNA. This rearrangement process enables a finite genome to produce an extremely high number of receptor combinations.

A complete BCR light chain is constructed from two gene segments, one of ~40κ or 30λ 'variable' (V) genes recombines to join one of 5κ or 4λ 'joining' (J) segments. The heavy chain is constructed independently from three gene segments by the splicing together of one of 27 'diversity' (D) segments with one of 6 J segments and one of ~42 V segments. This process is random, is driven by recombinase enzymes and can produce 10^{11} different BCR.

BCR can undergo further genetic modifications during an adaptive immune response. This process is called somatic mutation and results in an increased diversity of the B cell population. T cells cannot undergo somatic mutation, and all TCR rearrangement takes place in the thymus.

The TCR β chain rearranges first from the combination of one of 2 D gene segments with one of 52 V segments and one of 13 J segments. The α chain then rearranges and is produced by the combination of one ~70 V segments with one of 61 J genes to produce 10^{16} different αβ TCR.

This receptor diversity enables lymphocytes to respond specifically to a diverse world of pathogens and is the cornerstone of adaptive immune responses. Adaptive responses are not biased as the receptor rearrangement is a random process, so you can potentially recognize any antigen you are ever exposed to.

Receptor diversity generated by the recombination of multiple gene segments produces highly diverse lymphoid populations in each person, and this is referred to as your 'lymphocyte repertoire'.

Lysosomes Lysosomes are cytoplasmic granules containing hydrolytic enzymes involved in the digestion of phagocytosed material.

Macrophage Macrophages are large mononuclear phagocytic cells important in both innate and adaptive immunity. They are bone marrow derived (like all leukocytes) and develop from circulating monocytes that enter tissues where they differentiate into mature macrophages. Macrophages may have different names depending on the tissue they are found in (e.g. alveolar macrophages, kupffer cells, etc.). They can be identified by the expression of CD14 (LPS receptor) and they function to phagocytose pathogens, release pro-inflammatory cytokines (e.g. TNF-α and γIFN) and present antigen to T lymphocytes.

Major histocompatability complex (MHC). MHC molecules were first discovered for the important role they play in transplant rejection (hence the name histo and compatibility). MHC molecules are the most polymorphic genes in the human population. However, it is clear that these molecules play a central role in adaptive immune responses. They are peptide receptors—and cannot fold correctly in the absence of peptides. They 'present' these peptides to T cells.

There are two classes of MHC molecules: MHC class I and MHC class II. Their major difference is the source of peptide. MHC class I molecules bind to peptides of nine amino acids (these fit tightly into the groove) which are generated from within the cell. In contrast, MHC class II molecules bind to longer peptides (22–24 amino acids—these hang out of the groove) which enter the cell via the endosomal pathway (i.e. from the membrane/outside the cell). Each MHC molecule can bind 1000s of different peptides. Different MHC molecules will bind a different spectrum of peptides because they have distinct 'anchor residues'. For example, a certain class I MHC molecule will bind all peptides that have tyrosine at position 2 and a hydrophobic amino acid at position 9 (e.g. valine, isoleucine, leucine).

Mast cells Mast cells are bone marrow-derived cells found in connective tissue—mainly in the skin and mucosa. They possess numerous granules containing pro-inflammatory and toxic mediators. These include histamine, leukotrienes, pre-formed TNF alpha, fibroblast growth factor to name a few. They are characterized by expression of the high affinity Fc receptor for IgE which causes them to degranulate producing a local or systemic immediate hypersensitivity reaction. They promote inflammation following release of these anti-microbial and inflammatory mediators from granules and play an important role in defence against parasites and bacteria.

Mast cells also play an important role in allergic reactions, e.g. hay fever and asthma.

They can exist in a number of activation states, (a) resting, (b) sensitized (specific IgE bound to high affinity FcεR1) or (c) degranulating causing rapid release of preformed inflammatory mediators.

You can imagine them as cannons, situated at all our external barriers and ready to fire out their granular contents!

Memory cells Memory cells are differentiated lymphocytes (T and B) that have been clonally expanded following antigen exposure. They are easier to activate and mediate secondary immune responses following subsequent exposure to the same antigen.

In general, memory cells have higher levels of adhesion molecules and have a lower threshold for activation. When activated, they divide quicker and contain pre-formed effector molecules (e.g. perforin, cytokines). It is generally thought that memory T cells can be identified by the CD45RO isoform, whereas naive T cells that have not been exposed to their specific antigen express the longer CD45RA isoform.

Molecular mimicry Microbe-reactive T lymphocytes activated by recognition of microbial peptides presented by MHC molecules on antigen-presenting cells cross-react with MHC/self-peptide complexes, leading to autoimmunity. Microbe-reactive B lymphocytes activated by direct recognition of microbial antigen then cross-react with antigens expressed by host tissues, leading to autoimmunity.

Monoclonal antibody Monoclonal antibodies are antibodies produced by a single clone of B cells. Every single antibody has exactly the same specificity hence the term monoclonal. They are an invaluable tool in science because they can 'mark' a very specific structure. A Monoclonal antibody to CD14 will contain antibodies that only recognize one specific part of the CD14 molecule. Another monoclonal antibody to CD14 may recognize a different part of the CD14 molecule.

In normal immune responses, we make a 'polyclonal' response. If you are immunized with vaccine—then you will have lots of different antibodies that recognize the different cell surface structures present in that vaccine.

Glossary

Monocytes Monocytes are mononuclear bone marrow-derived cells that differentiate into tissue macrophages. They can be identified in Wright-Giemsa-stained blood smears by the presence of a kidney shaped nucleus. They can be identified immuno-histochemically by expression of CD14.

Naive lymphocytes Naive lymphocytes are those with BCR or TCR that have not undergone antigen recognition and therefore have not been activated or clonally expanded. Lymphocytes exiting primary lymphoid organs (bone marrow for B cells, thymus for T cells) are naive.

Naive lymphocytes express different cell surface markers and adhesion molecules to activated or memory ones, which affects their function. For example naive T cells can be identified by the expression of the higher molecular weight isoform of CD45—CD45RA and express l-selectin (which functions to bind MadCam-1 on high endothelial venules [HEV] on lymph nodes).

Natural Killer (NK) Cells NK cells are large granular lymphocytes that do not possess CD3 or a T cell receptor. They are able to recognize and destroy certain transformed and virally infected cells. Their killing ability is tightly regulated by inhibitory (MHC molecules) and activating receptors, or can be induced by antibodies (antibody-dependent cellular cytotoxicity ADCC).

NK cells induce target cell apoptosis following release of perforin and granzymes.

Necrosis Cell death stimulated by chemical or physical injury (external factors) and results in release of cellular debris and local damage. It generally leads to inflammation.

Neutralization The process of inhibiting the infectivity of a virus or the toxicity of a toxin molecule are said to neutralize them. Antibodies with this property are known as neutralizing antibodies and it leads to viral inactivation.

Neutrophil Also referred to as polymorphonuclear cells (PMN) or granulocyte.

Neutrophils are short-lived, bone marrow-derived cells (half-life 6–12 h) and are the most common white blood cells. They are identified by their characteristic multi-lobed nuclei. They are typically the first cell to reach tissue following injury or infection. They function to internalize pathogens and destroy them by phagocytosis. They also release a number of toxic mediators (e.g. neutrophil elastase) that contribute to tissue damage. They can undergo an unusual form of cell death whereby they release nuclear material (DNA, histones, and granular proteins) extracellularly which can trap exogenous bacteria in a process known as NETosis.

You will have seen neutrophils after an injury/skin infection (yellow-green pus). You can imagine them as the foot soldiers of your innate responses, rushing into battle when the outer defences have been breached.

NF-κβ NF-κβ is a transcription factor found in all cells which plays a key role in the activation of immune response genes. The NF-κβ pathway is activated by pattern recognition receptors (PRR) and proinflammatory cytokines (e.g. IL1 and TNFα). The inactivated form exists in the cytoplasm in combination with inhibitors (e.g. I-κβ). The activated molecule (made up of a subunit of RelA and p50 or RelB and p52) translocates to the nucleus and binds to immune response genes which can activate adaptive immune responses. It plays a key role in inflammation, but also affects a wide range of biological processes (e.g. growth, development and apoptosis).

Normal adult blood cell counts

Cell Type	Cells/l (normal range)	%
Red blood cells	$3.8–5.9 \times 10^{12}$	
Platelets	$1.5–3.5 \times 10^{11}$	
White blood cells (WBC):	**7.3×10^9**	
Polymorphonuclear cells		
– Neutrophils	$1.8–7.7 \times 10^9$	**~60% of WBC**
– Eosinophils	$0–0.45 \times 10^9$	**~2.7% of WBC**
– Basophils	$0–0.2 \times 10^9$	**~0.5% of WBC**

Mononuclear cells		
– Monocytes	0–0.8×10^9	~**4% of WBC**
– Lymphocytes:	1.6–4.8×10^9	~**24% of WBC**
consisting of –		
– B cells		10–15% of lymphocytes
– CD4+ T cells		50–60% of lymphocytes
– CD8+ T cells		20–25% of lymphocytes
– Natural Killer (NK) cells		~10% of lymphocytes

Nuclear factor of activated T cells (NFAT) NFAT plays a key role in T cell biology. It exists in the cytoplasm in a phosphorylated state, dephosphorylates under the action of calcineurin (Ca^2+ activated) and enters the nucleus where it binds the IL-2 promoter. The immunosuppressive drugs Cyclosporin A and Tacrolimus (FK506) block calcineurin, thereby inhibiting NFAT activation and IL-2 gene transcription. This has a profound effect on T cell proliferation and explains the success of these agents to block immune responses, e.g. transplant rejection.

Nuclear factors The transcription of genes is initiated and regulated through the actions of nuclear factors and results in the production of messenger RNA which is transferred to the cytoplasm and serves as the template for protein synthesis. There are many different nuclear factors that co-ordinate and control this process.

Opsonization Opsonization is the alteration of the surface of a pathogen (or particle) so that it can be ingested by phagocytes. Typically, the pathogen is coated with a self protein (e.g. complement proteins). Phagocytes have receptors for this protein, and can therefore bind to, and ingest, the pathogen more efficiently.

Paracrine Paracrine effects are those produced by one cell and exerted on another nearby cell. For example, a soluble mediator produced by one cell binds to a receptor on another cell nearby and exerts a biological effect.

Pathogen Any organism capable of causing disease and damage when it infects a host is a pathogen. They are typically viruses, bacteria, yeasts or parasites.

Pathogen-associated molecular pattern (PAMP) Innate responses are directed against common microbial structures found on pathogens. These molecular patterns serve as 'antigens' to pattern recognition molecules of the innate defences and stimulate inflammation.

Pattern recognition receptors (PRR) Pattern Recognition Receptors or molecules bind to Pathogen-Associated Molecular Patterns (PAMPs). There are many examples, some are listed below:

Protein family	Site	Example	Ligand	Function
Collectin	Humoral	Mannan binding lectin (MBL)	bacterial and viral carbohydrates	Opsonization c' activation
Cellular	Macrophage, DC	Macrophage c-type lectin	GalNAc receptor	Induces macrophage killing
	Macrophage, DC	Macrophage mannose receptor	Terminal mannose	Phagocytosis
	Macrophage, DC	DEC205	Terminal mannose	Phagocytosis

Leucine rich proteins	Macrophage, epithelial cells	CD14	LPS	Activation – signals to cell
	B cells	TOLL-like	Unknown CHO	Activation – B cell growth
	Macrophage (some)	Macrophage receptor with collagenous structure (MARCO)	Bacterial cell walls	Phagocytosis
Pentraxins	Plasma proteins	C-Reactive Protein	Phospatidyl choline	Opsonization, activate complement cascade
	Plasma proteins	Serum amyloid P	Bacterial cell walls	Opsonization, activate complement cascade
Lipid transferase	Plasma protein	LBP	LPS, LS	Bind LPS and transfer to CD14

Perforin Perforin is a protein present in the cytolytic granules of CTL and NK cells which polymerizes to form a pore in the membrane of a target cell (like C9 of the membrane attack complex of the complement system). This allows proteolytic granzymes access to the cytoplasm of the target cell.

Phagocytosis To consume by enveloping and digesting. From the Greek Phagein—to eat. It is the process of engulfing bacteria or other particles into special organelles within the cell called phagosomes. These quickly merge with cytoplasmic granules that contain a formidable array of chemicals with anti-bacterial activity. This arsenal of antibacterial agents includes lysozyme, lactoferrin, proteolytic enzymes and a family of anti-microbial peptides called defensins. The fusion of the granules with the phagosome exposes the bacteria to these toxic compounds and results in bacterial elimination.

Phenotype This is defined as the sum of total 'visible' traits which characterize members of a group. The phenotype of a leukocyte is the cell surface molecules it possesses.

For example, if you know that all macrophages and monocytes express the LPS receptor, CD14. You can then phenotype a group of cells (e.g. in a tissue, or blood) by staining them with an antibody to CD14. You know any positive cells must be monocytes/macrophages since they express CD14

Plasma cell Plasma cells are differentiated B lymphocytes and are generally found in organized lymphoid tissue. They secrete antibody molecules of the same specificity as the BCR, however the class of the antibody molecules (IgM, IgG, IgA, IgE), and therefore the function of the antibody, can change depending on the stimulation received.

Polymorphic Genetic polymorphism means that a certain gene locus can have numerous variants or 'alleles'. Many genes are polymorphic (e.g. cytokine genes).

However, the most polymorphic gene in the body is the MHC. There are multiple alleles of MHC class I and class II genes in the population. For more information, visit http://www.ebi.ac.uk/imgt/hla/. It is therefore unlikely that anyone has the same six class I MHC molecules and same six class II MHC molecules as you, great if you want to make a diverse immune response, not so great if you need a transplant!

Primary immune response Is the initial adaptive immune response to a novel antigen.

It involves the activation of naive lymphocytes and leads to the generation of an immune response and memory. Responses take time to generate (generally 7–10 days), and are of a lesser magnitude than secondary responses.

Pyroptosis An inflammatory form of cell death which leads to inflammation. It has been associated with the activation of the enzyme capsase 1.

Reactive nitrogen species (RNS) Toxic, free radical and other forms of molecular nitrogen which have an antimicrobial effect. The most important example is Nitric Oxide (NO) produced by the action of inducible NO synthase during phagocytosis.

Reactive oxygen species (ROS) Toxic, free radical and other forms of molecular oxygen which have an antimicrobial effect. Examples include Hydrogen peroxide (H_2O_2), the superoxide radical (O_2^-) and the destructive hydroxyl radical (.OH). This contributes to microbial killing during phagocytosis.

Recombination activating genes (RAG) 1 and 2 RAG1 and 2 encode proteins essential to the recombination of BCR and TCR immunoglobulin gene segments. They drive the diversity of lymphoid cell populations by mediating V(D)J joining.

Lack of functional RAG results in a failure to produce mature recombined BCR and TCR, leading to a lack of mature B and T cells and a severe combined immunodeficiency (SCID).

Restriction factors Anti-viral proteins that limit or restrict viral replication.

Rheumatoid arthritis A chronic autoimmune inflammatory disease affecting primarily the joints.

Rheumatoid factor (RF) This is an IgM antibody specific to determinants on IgG found in 60–80% of patients with rheumatoid arthritis. However it is also found in other autoimmune diseases (e.g. scleroderma, Still's disease, Sjörgen syndrome and systemic lupus erythematosa) and in some infections.

Secondary immune response Is the adaptive immune response to an antigen to which you have been previously exposed.

It involves the activation of memory lymphocytes and leads to a rapid, escalating response against the specific antigen.

Secondary responses are quicker and stronger than primary responses (generally evident in 2–3 days).

Selectins Selectins are a family of adhesion molecules which bind to carbohydrate (CHO) groups on specific glycoproteins and mucin-containing molecules. It is thought that the selectins can bind to a number of sugar ligands with low affinity. Selectin–CHO bonds form and break as leukocytes roll along blood vessel walls.

Selectins contain a calcium-dependent (C-type) lectin domain at their N-terminus.

L-selectin (CD62L) is expressed on leukocytes.

P-selectin (CD62P) and E-selectin (CD62E) are expressed by endothelial cells and platelets.

Somatic recombination DNA recombination that takes place in somatic cells. This is distinct from the DNA recombination that takes place during meiosis.

Spleen The spleen is a secondary lymphoid organ containing red and white pulp. Red pulp is involved with removing senescent (old) red blood cells. White pulp contains lymphoid cells that respond to pathogens delivered to the spleen by the blood.

T cell antigen receptor (TCR) Expressed by T lymphocytes and composed of a dimeric molecule which comprises a rearranged αβ chain, or more rarely a γδ chain.

αβ TCR recognize MHC/peptide complexes on other cells and cannot recognize pathogens directly. They are therefore MHC restricted. This is a consequence of positive selection in the thymus. αβ T cells are the most common and constitute about 95% of the T cell population. Current understanding of T lymphocytes is based on those with αβ TCR.

γδ TCR are found close to epithelial cells, particularly in the gut. They show a more unrestricted recognition and may recognize antigens in a manner more related to antibodies than αβ T cells. Their function is unknown, although they have been proposed to play a role in tumour surveillance, oral tolerance and early protection against microbes. For example, they have the ability to bind to glycolipids and heat shock proteins found in mycobacterial cell walls and products (PPD, purified protein derivative).

Glossary

(TGFβ) Transforming Growth Factor beta (TGFβ) is a multi-functional cytokine that plays a role in development, extracellular matrix degradation and synthesis, epithelial/fibroblast cell growth and differentiation, monocyte chemotaxis, carcinogenesis and angiogenesis. It is typically regarded as an anti-inflammatory and pro-fibrotic cytokine.

It is tightly regulated and secreted as a large latent complex (a dimer of TGFβ pro-peptide complexed with a latency associated protein [LAP] and latent TGFβ binding protein [LTBP]) which can bind the ECM. TGFβ therefore needs to be activated prior to activity by proteases (e.g. plasmin).

TGFβ can be produced by a wide range of cell types including lymphocytes (often those associated with tolerance, e.g. Treg), macrophages, platelets and epithelial cells.

Mucosal tissues in particular contain high concentrations of TGFβ which can modify the function of lymphocytes and their expression of surface molecules (e.g. TGFβ upregulates expression of CD103 or αE the mucosal integrin on lymphocytes, the ligand for e-cadherin expressed by epithelial cells. This probably functions to retain lymphocytes in the intra-epithelial compartment.)

Thymus A primary lymphoid organ and site of T lymphocyte development. It is most active in children and undergoes atrophy in adults.

T lymphocyte (or T cell) T lymphocytes are a subset of lymphocytes defined by their development in the thymus and expression of a T cell receptor (TCR; alpha beta or gamma delta heterodimers). T lymphocytes do not directly recognize pathogens, but MHC/peptide complexes expressed on antigen-presenting cells (APC).

T lymphocytes can be characterized by the expression of CD3 (part of the TCR complex) and can be subdivided into two major classes by the expression of either CD4 or CD8. CD4+ T lymphocytes recognize class II MHC/peptide complexes whereas CD8+ T lymphocytes are restricted to class I MHC/peptide complexes.

They play a key role in adaptive immune responses and function to either produce cytokines (CD4+) or kill infected/transformed self cells (CD8+).

TNFα (TNF alpha) Tumour necrosis factor alpha (TNFα) is a pro-inflammatory cytokine produced by mast cells/eosinophils, macrophages and natural killer cells. It modifies the biological response of many cells and exerts multiple effects. TNFα contributes to inflammation and stimulates the acute phase response (together with IL-1, IL-6, for which reason it is also referred to as an 'endogenous pyrogen' since it raises body temperature). Clinically, it contributes to septic shock (during acute inflammation) and weight loss (during chronic inflammation).

TNFα has been implicated in the pathology of a wide range of chronic inflammatory conditions including arthritis and inflammatory bowel disease. Interestingly, anti-TNF therapy has been more successful than any other cytokine treatment clinically (e.g. IL-1ra, anti-IL-6r, IL-10, IL-11, IL-4, TGFβ)—indicating the dominant role of this cytokine in inflammatory cascade. Anti-TNFα antibodies are used to treat rheumatoid arthritis (in combination with methotrexate) and Crohn's disease.

Toll-like receptors (TLR) A family of highly conserved innate receptors that lead to the upregulation of immune response genes. All members of this family are type 1 membrane proteins.

Toll pathway A universal pathway that leads to the activation immune response genes in all host defence systems. Characterized by the transcription factor NF-κβ.

Transformation Transformation is the change that a normal cell makes when it becomes malignant. It is generally a permanent change involving a genetic mutation.

Normal cells have a finite life span and eventually die. Growth is dysregulated in transformed cells so that they do not die and have an infinite life span.

Tumour A group of cells which have lost normal control over cell division and so proliferate inappropriately.

Index

A

acquired immunodeficiency syndrome (AIDS) 93, 99, 101, 102, 117
see also human immunodeficiency virus
activating receptors (ARs) 76
activation of adaptive immune system 48–64
acute local inflammation 4–6
acute phase protein 3, 7, 8, 36, 123
acute rejection (AR), transplantation 115
acute systemic inflammation 6–8
adaptive effector mechanisms 79–89
adaptive immunity 1, 2, 3, 10–15, 123
 activation 48–64
 diversity 18
 and inflammasomes 40
 lymph nodes 19
 mannose receptor 36
 mucosa-associated lymphoid organs 22
 and NFκβ 39
 primary immune response 11–13
 recognition 33, 34, 41, 42–8
 secondary immune responses 13–15
 secondary lymphoid organs 19
 T cells 23
 thymus removal 19
 transplant rejection 111, 114
Addison's disease 104, 106
adhesion molecules 5, 6, 123
affinity maturation 46–7, 123
agammaglobulinaemias 96–7
age related macular degeneration 72
agglutination 81, 123
AIDS *see* acquired immunodeficiency syndrome

alarmins 78, 123
 see also damage associated molecular patterns
alemtuzumab 120
allergen 107, 123
allergy 23, 24, 59
 see also hypersensitivity
allograft 111
alpha-1-antitrypsin 8
alpha acid glycoprotein 8
alphafetoprotein (AFP) 118
ALPS (autoimmune lymphoproliferative syndrome) 97
alternative pathway, complement activation 70, 71, 72, 74, 86
alveolar macrophages 24
anaphylaxis 107, 108, 109
anaphylatoxins 71, 73, 123
anergy 57, 123
angioedema, hereditary 73
angiogenesis 116
ankylosing spondylitis 105, 106
Annexin V 117
anthrax 14
antibiotics 94
antibodies 45, 81, 124
 as effector molecules 81–8
 blood group antigens 109
 deficiencies 94, 98
 primary immune response 11
 protein structure 81, 82
 transplant rejection 115, 116
antibody dependent cellular cytotoxicity (ADCC) 67, 86, 87, 123
antigen presenting cells (APC) 15, 49, 51, 124
 class II MHC 43
 cytotoxic T lymphocytes 88
 dendritic cells 25
 lymph nodes 20
 primary immune response 11
 T cell activation 54
antigen receptors 44, 124

antigens 13, 25, 124
 lymphocyte receptors 42
 presentation 49–53
 primary immune response 11
 secondary lymphoid organs 19
 tumours 117–18
anti-histamines 109
anti-inflammatory cytokines 116
anti-inflammatory drugs 109
antimicrobial peptides 69
antiphospholipid syndrome 105
anti-retroviral drugs 103
anti-tumour immune responses 24
anti-viral immune responses 24, 41
AP-1 58
APECED (autoimmune polyendocrinopathy candidiasis ectodermal dystrophy) 97
apoptosis 78, 124
 B cell antigen receptors 16
 cytotoxic T lymphocytes 89, 90
 T cells 48
 thymus 17
arthus reaction 110
asthma 23, 24
autoantibodies 105, 105–6
autocrine 27, 124
autograft 111
autoimmune hepatitis 105
autoimmune lymphoproliferative syndrome (ALPS) 97
autoimmune pernicious anaemia 105
autoimmune polyendocrinopathy candidiasis ectodermal dystrophy (APECED) 97
autoimmune regulator (AIRE) 97
autoimmunity 93, 104–7
 DiGeorge's syndrome 98
 hypersensitivity 110
 thymus 18
autoinflammatory diseases 97–8

Index

Index